RAPIDZAP

AUTOMATED DEFIBRILLATION

RAPIDZAP
AUTOMATED DEFIBRILLATION

Judy Reid Graves, R.N., M.A., EMT-P

Douglas Austin, Jr., EMT-P

Richard O. Cummins, M.D., M.P.H., M.Sc.

BRADY
Prentice Hall Career & Technology
Englewood Cliffs, New Jersey 07632

Library of Congress Cataloging-in-Publication Data

Graves, Judy Reid.
Rapidzap : automated defibrillation / Judy Reid Graves, Douglas Austin, Richard O. Cummins.
p. cm.
"A Brady book."
Bibliography: p.
ISBN 0-89303-813-X
1. Ventricular fibrillation--Treatment. 2. Electric countershock. 3. Defibrillators. I. Austin, Douglas. II. Cummins, Richard O. III. Title.
RC685.V43G72 1989
616.1'280645--dc19
89-30264
CIP

Editorial/production supervision and
interior design: *Ellen Denning*
Cover design: *Lundgren Graphics, Ltd.*
Manufacturing buyer: *Robert Anderson*

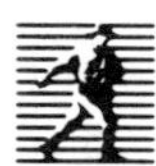

Prentice-Hall, Inc.
A Paramount Communications Company
Englewood Cliffs, New Jersey 07632

NOTICE:

It is the intent of the authors and publishers that this textbook be used as part of a formal automated defibrillation course taught by a qualified instructor. The care procedures presented here represent accepted practices in the United States. They are not offered as a standard of care. EMT-level emergency care is to be performed under the authority and guidance of a licensed physician. It is the reader's responsibility to know and follow local care protocols as provided by the medical advisors directing the system to which he or she belongs. Also, it is the reader's responsibility to stay informed of emergency care procedure changes.

Printed in the United States of America

10 9 8 7 6 5

ISBN 0-89303-813-X

PRENTICE-HALL INTERNATIONAL (UK) LIMITED, *London*
PRENTICE-HALL OF AUSTRALIA PTY. LIMITED, *Sydney*
PRENTICE-HALL CANADA INC. *Toronto*
PRENTICE-HALL HISPANOAMERICANA, S.A., *Mexico*
PRENTICE-HALL OF INDIA PRIVATE LIMITED, *New Delhi*
PRENTICE-HALL OF JAPAN, INC., *Tokyo*
SIMON & SCHUSTER ASIA PTE. LTD., *Singapore*
EDITORA PRENTICE-HALL DO BRASIL, LTDA., *Rio de Janeiro*

CONTENTS

FOREWORD

Every day nearly 1000 Americans die of heart attack before reaching a hospital. Many others die of accidents such as drowning, electrocution, and suffocation that interrupt normal breathing and heartbeat. The primary killer in these instances is a chaotic disturbance of normal heart rhythm known as ventricular fibrillation. This condition causes death from cardiac arrest within minutes unless rapid treatment is given.

Fortunately, we now have both the knowledge and equipment to reverse ventricular fibrillation and prevent death. Small, lightweight, easy-to-use, computerized heart treatment devices called automated external defibrillators have been used successfully by all levels of emergency response personnel as well as trained citizen responders. These machines automatically detect ventricular fibrillation and deliver one or more electrical shocks to restart normal heart rhythm.

Numerous studies have proven the effectiveness of this approach. Today's challenge is not to study but to implement. We must place this equipment in the hands of all rescuers who routinely arrive first on the scene of cardiac arrest.

The most ambitious effort to date has been the initiation of a rapid defibrillation project by the Emergency Medical Services Committee of the International Association of Fire Chiefs (IAFC) in 1986. The goal of the project was significant reduction of the loss of life from cardiac arrest by encouraging the placement of automated defibrillators on all fire apparatus in the nation's 32,000 fire departments rather than only on ambulance and rescue units.

An IAFC demonstration project was conducted in Eugene and Springfield, Oregon (population 160,000). All firefighters were trained to use automated defibrillators and every fire engine was equipped. Survival increased by 18 percent in the first year. The project was nicknamed "RapidZap" by Springfield Fire Chief Don Herschel, and the IAFC project was given birth. Multiple-unit first-response defibrillation projects are now operating in Seattle/King County, Washington; Dallas, Texas; Salt Lake City, Utah; Jacksonville and Tampa, Florida; Lincoln, Nebraska; Denver, Colorado; Des Moines and Cedar Rapids, Iowa; Rochester, Minnesota; Eugene and Springfield, Oregon; and many other cities of all sizes.

Another issue of growing concern is addressed by the RapidZap project—firefighter safety. According to the National Fire Protection Association, heart attack has been the leading killer of firefighters for many years, causing nearly half of the on-duty deaths of both paid and volunteer personnel. Many millions of dollars have been spent to improve safety through safer firefighting personal clothing and other equipment; however, there has been no sustained decrease in firefighter deaths since 1982. Little attention has been given to the safety benefits of placing automated defibrillators on all apparatus. Already, firefighters' lives have been saved because a shock was administered immediately following a heart attack by fellow firefighters riding on the same engine. This new information may well pave the way for a systematic reduction in firefighter deaths.

As suggested by the name "RapidZap," speed is the all-important factor in saving the life of a cardiac arrest victim. Each minute that passes means that the victim is several percent less likely to survive. If we are to beat the clock, we must view anything that delays rapid delivery of a lifesaving shock as an obstacle that must be removed. From the call for help to the arrival of trained personnel, everything must move quickly. Citizens must be taught to phone 911 or other emergency number without delay; the call must be promptly and effeciently processed; and responders must arrive quickly and deliver the shock immediately upon arrival. CPR is still important, but ultimately its only purpose is to buy a few extra minutes to get the defibrillator to the victim.

Public information and education are important to gain the necessary support for implementation. RapidZap promotion packages are now available to help overcome various problems and raise funds for training and equipment.

The ultimate frontier may lie well beyond equipping all fire apparatus with automated defibrillators. In the case of some remote areas, sheriff officers, state police, or forest service personnel could be equipped. In large buildings, to prevent delay, security guards could be trained to use the equipment and defibrillators placed in several locations. Golf courses, resorts, and other health or fitness centers, where there is a greater risk of cardiac arrest or a delayed response, should also be considered. Expansion of rapid defibrillation will ultimately lead to the development of even smaller, lighter, and less expensive defibrillators. Eventually, high-risk heart patients may enjoy activities never before possible by carrying a personal defibrillator wherever they go.

This textbook is expertly written to benefit a vast potential audience now and in the future. Its authors possess a unique combination of skills and experience—from research, analysis, and training, to quality assurance and hands-on experience with citizens, first responders, EMTs, and paramedics. It will meet the needs of the automated defibrillation student, while assisting trainers, medical directors, and administrators in establishing a solid program. Please join me in welcoming the opportunity to participate in what has already become one of the most significant advances in public safety in this century!

DENNIS M. MURPHY

Chairman, RapidZap Project
Emergency Medical Services Committee
International Association of Fire Chiefs

Division Chief
Springfield Department of Fire & Life Safety
Springfield, Oregon

PREFACE

Who should read this book? The principle of early defibrillation states that the first person to respond to someone in cardiac arrest should be equipped with a defibrillator. This book is intended for all emergency personnel who are learning about automated external defibrillators as part of an early defibrillation training program. This book serves as the textbook for your course. The book is also written for the training officers of EMS or fire services programs interested in the now widely endorsed concept of early prehospital defibrillation. You may be considering whether to start such program, how it should be set up, and especially how to maintain it and assure ongoing high quality. This book will help you make such decisions and guide you in getting started. The detailed automated defibrillator curriculum should be particularly helpful. This book will also help any physician who has agreed to become the medical director for an early defibrillation program. This book gives you a discussion of the pros and cons for many of the decisions you will have to make: details of the standing orders, contents for the training classes, and how to maintain medical control.

We have omitted details of the operation of the currently available automated defibrillators for several important reasons. New automated defibrillators are being developed and will soon reach the market. Specific operation material in this book would soon be out of date. Manufacturers have produced excellent operational manuals and literature that can be distributed at the training classes. This handbook can be read quickly the evening before the course and can later serve as a ready reference. Finally, a small book is inexpensive and can thus be purchased for each participant in the program.

A note on terminology. In this book we use the term "automated external defibrillators/defibrillation" as a generic term to refer to all external defibrillators that include a rhythm analysis system. Some companies manufacture devices which they call "fully" automatic, and others use the term "semiautomatic" or "automatic advisory." We indicate when we refer to the defibrillators manufactured by specific companies. Otherwise, the terms "automated external defibrillators" and "defibrillation" are used only in a generic sense and do not refer to the products of specific companies.

In addition, when we use the term "EMS rescuers" it applies to all emergency personnel who have been authorized by a medical control authority to participate in an early defibrillation program. This includes emergency medical technicians (EMT-Ds), "first responders" who have completed the Department of Transportation 40-hour first-responder course, and firefighters who participate in a RapidZap program. It also includes policemen, security personnel, highway patrolmen, airline flight attendents, and other rescuers who respond to people in cardiac arrest and who have been authorized to use automated external defibrillators.

Products described. This book contains photographs, some technical information, and proposed treatment protocols for a number of automated external defibrillators. No endorsement of any product is intended, nor should one be inferred.

National standards for early defibrillation. An important development took place in April 1986 when the National Council of State Emergency Medical Services Training Coordinators (NCSEMSTC) sponsored a seminar on standards for EMT defibrillation programs. Completion of these national standards is in its final stages. The authors of this book participated in this standard setting seminar; all recommendations in this book are consistent with these standards.

Royalty distribution. All royalties from the sale of this work go to the Center for Evaluation of Emergency Medical Services, Emergency Medical Services Division, Seattle–King County Department of Public Health, Seattle, Washington.

JUDY REID GRAVES
DOUGLAS AUSTIN, JR.
RICHARD O. CUMMINS

ACKNOWLEDGMENTS

We acquired a great deal of our understanding and experience with automated external defibrillation during the conduct of a controlled clinical trial of automated external defibrillators used by emergency medical technicians (JAMA 1987;257:1605–1610). This trial was generously supported by a grant from the National Center for Health Services Research (HS-05174) and a grant from the Cardiac Resuscitator Corporation, Portland, Oregon. In addition, the Physio-Control Corporation of Redmond, Washington, and the Laerdal Medical Corporation of Armonk, New York, have graciously provided us with detailed information about their automated external defibrillators.

This book was the product of numerous conversations and shared experiences with many people, in particular, Mickey Eisenberg, Susan Damon, Cindy Hambly, Don Sorenson, Ken Stults, Michael Copass, Dennis Murphy, and Arthur Kellerman. We express our special thanks to the many emergency medical technicians of King County, Washington, who for over six years have used automated defibrillators to snatch precious life from the gaping jaws of death.

RAPIDZAP

AUTOMATED DEFIBRILLATION

Chapter 1

THE IMPORTANCE OF EARLY DEFIBRILLATION

A. THE BATTLE AGAINST SUDDEN CARDIAC DEATH BY THE FIRST RESPONDER

In most places in the United States, emergency medical services first responders are the first emergency personnel to reach a person who has collapsed in cardiac arrest. They initiate two-rescuer CPR and provide better cerebral and coronary blood flow and oxygenation than most bystanders. But that's all. First responders must either await the arrival of paramedics or "scoop and run" with the patient to the nearest emergency facility. Approximately 60 percent of out-of-hospital cardiac arrest patients are discovered to be in the cardiac rhythm called *ventricular fibrillation* when emergency personnel arrive at their side (see Figure 1–1). Unless an electrical shock is rapidly delivered to that person's heart, the heart will continue to weaken, all heart action will cease, and restoration of an effective heartbeat will be impossible.

In many EMS and fire service systems in the United States and in other countries, emergency personnel have been equipped with defibrillators and trained to shock ventricular fibrillation within 1 to 2 minutes of arriving at the patient's side. The purpose of training these responders to defibrillate was to provide the earliest possible defibrillation. In several locations first responders and EMTs have achieved a survival rate for patients in ventricular fibrillation comparable to that achieved by paramedics. EMTs and EMS first responders find them-

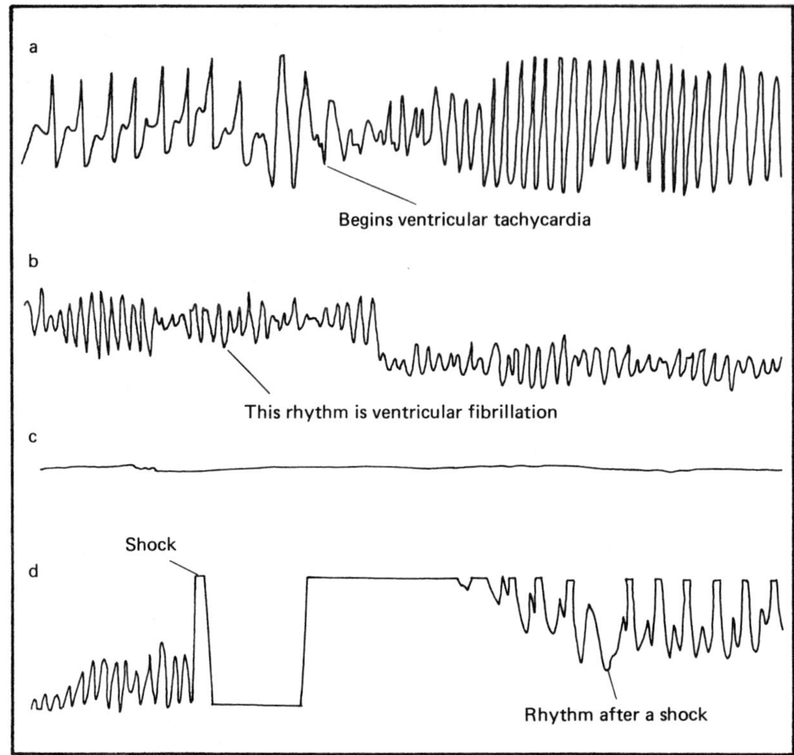

Figure 1–1 Rhythms of the dying heart. Heart attack produces abnormal cardiac rhythms that can be analyzed on the ECG monitor. (a) Early cardiac disturbance is ventricular tachycardia. (b) Ventricular tachycardia often is followed promptly by ventricular fibrillation, a sign of ineffective cardiac function. (c) If untreated, asystole, or cardiac standstill, will occur. (d) If an electrical shock is applied to the heart during the time of ventricular fibrillation, normal electrical activity can be restored and effective cardiac contractions can resume. (Reproduced with permission from American Academy of Orthopaedic Surgeons, *Emergency Care and Transportation of the Sick and Injured,* 4th ed. © 1987.)

selves in a peculiar position. They have long been known for being able to respond quickly and to do effective CPR. But whether or not that patient survives an out-of-hospital cardiac arrest depends on additional factors. These factors have to do with both the patient and the EMS system. A person is most likely to be rescued from a cardiac arrest if:

1. The event is observed by someone who calls for help quickly.
2. The emergency medical service personnel respond quickly.

3. CPR is started *early* by family members, bystanders, EMTs, or first responders.
4. Defibrillation is performed as close as possible to the time of the cardiac arrest.
5. The patient receives additional advanced life support either from paramedics in the field or from physicians at a hospital.
6. The patient's heart disease is not inevitably terminal.

The concept of rapid defibrillation has evolved as a means to achieve point 4—early defibrillation. The emergency rescuer, so close to the time and location of sudden death for most patients, is unable to do anything but good CPR. We know it is application of shocks to the heart that can restore the heartbeat and make a life or death difference. EMTs, fire service rescuers, and first responders armed with defibrillators are participating in the most exciting new development in prehospital care.

B. THE IMPACT ON DEATH RATES

The world's most effective emergency medical service programs have made early defibrillation a building block to their success. Present national survival rates from cardiac arrest are 3 to 5 percent—roughly 1 of 20 cardiac arrest patients survive. The survival rates in EMS systems that include early defibrillation are 20 to 25 percent (or 1 in 4 people). Addition of rapid first-responder and EMT defibrillation to systems without this service should increase the number of people who survive sudden cardiac death.

C. IS RAPID EARLY DEFIBRILLATION RIGHT FOR YOU?

We think an early defibrillation program is right for communities in which the following exist:

1. First rescuer response times are short, less than 15 minutes. Patients treated more than 15 minutes after they arrest have a poor chance of survival.
2. Most cardiac arrests in the area are witnessed. The best reported survival rate for unwitnessed arrests is less than 2 percent.
3. Bystanders begin CPR often and quickly, within 4 minutes of the collapse. CPR started after that time has markedly reduced effectiveness.
4. The community is large enough to expect one out-of-hospital car-

diac arrest per year. This means about 1000 people. This recommendation of one arrest per year is really a suggestion, not a requirement. It is our rough estimate of what an early defibrillation program needs to support skills, maintain interest and enthusiasm, and leave a sense of money well spent. A community with an unusual age distribution, such as many elderly people, may experience even more cardiac arrests.

5. Similarly, advanced life support, in the form of personnel or nearby emergency facilities, should not be too far away. It should be available within a reasonable time—less than 15 minutes is best—after a patient is defibrillated.

Lack of some of these features, such as advanced life-support personnel, will prevent a Rapid Zap program from achieving maximum effectiveness. Nevertheless, in virtually all communities a possibility remains that a Rapid Zap program will save lives. Emergency medical personnel should view the criteria listed above as rough guidelines to estimate how effective an early defibrillation program could be in their communities. We hope that some communities will realize immediately that an early defibrillation program is not for them. Similarly, other communities will see at once that such a program is exactly what is needed to save more lives in their community.

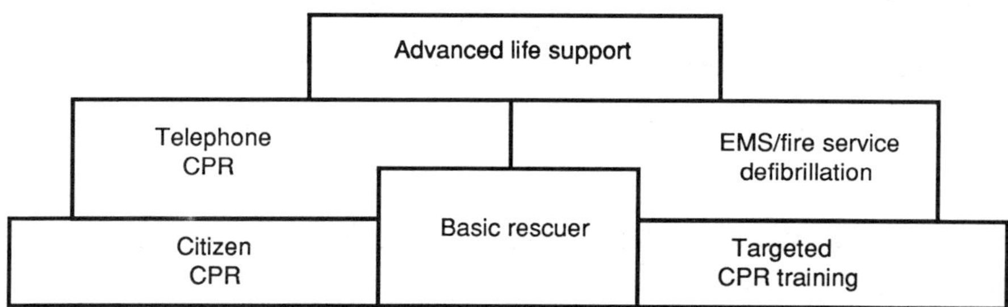

Figure 1–2 Hierarchy of emergency medical services, including early defibrillation, for the management of sudden cardiac death in the community. [Adapted from M. Eisenberg, L. Bergner, and A. Hallstrom, *Sudden Cardiac Death in the Community* (Praeger Publishers, New York, 1984.), p. 141. Copyright © 1984 by Praeger Publishers. Used with permission.]

Chapter 2

THE DYING HEART

A. INTRODUCTION

Heart disease is the greatest killer of adults in the United States. Over 700,000 die each year from heart disease in the United States. Of these people, half die in the hospital, but the other half die outside the hospital: in the home, in places of work, and in the streets. These out-of-hospital deaths have been a major force behind the development of emergency medical services, first responders, and EMT and paramedic programs. In the early 1970s research demonstrated that if advanced medical skills were taken directly to a person collapsed in cardiac arrest, lives could be saved.

B. THE PHYSIOLOGY OF CORONARY HEART DISEASE

A great deal of scientific and medical attention has been devoted to defining the causes of cardiac arrest. Although much is known, there is still much that needs to be understood. Sudden cardiac death most often occurs in people in their 50s and 60s, although it may occur less commonly in persons who are 30 to 40. It is three times more common in men than in women. People who have sudden cardiac arrest usually have underlying atherosclerotic heart disease: hardening of the arteries. Atherosclerosis is a slow, progressive disease that begins in teenagers in the United States, and continues slowly into adulthood. The walls of the arteries become thickened with deposits of fatty substances such as cholesterol. As the arteries become narrowed, the blood supply to various parts of the heart is reduced. If the narrowing becomes too great and the vessel becomes blocked, that portion of the body that is supplied by the artery is severely damaged. When the arteries of the heart are involved and one becomes blocked, the portion of the heart supplied by that artery is damaged. This is what is known as a *myocardial infarction* ("an MI"), or heart attack.

Cardiac Muscle Death

In a heart attack a block occurs in one of the arteries directly supplying blood to the heart muscle. When the blood supply becomes blocked, the heart muscle begins to die. If the heart muscle is starved of oxygen and nutrients, the muscle cannot function properly. Damaged muscle releases acids, which cause an area of irritability. This in turn causes the heart's pumping rhythm to become very abnormal. If the abnormal rhythm is ventricular fibrillation, the heart can no longer pump effectively and no blood is pumped out to the body. This is called a *cardiac arrest.*

Electrical Death

Another way in which sudden cardiac arrest may occur is through electrical death. In this situation a heart attack, in which a portion of the heart muscle becomes damaged, does not occur. Instead, for reasons that are not well understood, the heart's normal rhythm suddenly turns into a fatal rhythm (in most cases, ventricular fibrillation). This sudden change from a normal rhythm to a fatal rhythm also results in sudden cardiac arrest. Although persons with sudden cardiac arrest have underlying atherosclerosis, only one out of three has actually had a blocked coronary artery with muscle damage. The rest have had their arrest produced by an electrical disturbance. The result, however, is the same. A heart that was normally pumping blood to the body suddenly stops because of the disturbance in rhythm, and unless advanced cardiac care is provided quickly, the person will die.

C. RISK FACTORS FOR SUDDEN CARDIAC ARREST

There are many risk factors that contribute to the development of atherosclerosis and thus make a person a prime candidate for a heart attack and a cardiac arrest. These include:

1. Persons with a family history of early heart disease are more likely to develop atherosclerosis. Having a father or mother or aunt or uncle who died of heart disease before the age of 50 is a particularly strong risk factor.
2. Cigarette smoking is the next-strongest risk factor for sudden cardiac death.
3. High blood pressure that is not controlled with medication is a strong factor that contributes to the development of heart disease.
4. A high-fat diet with high levels of cholesterol causes the process of atherosclerosis to progress more rapidly.
5. Diabetes is a risk factor for premature heart disease, particularly diabetes that must be treated with insulin injections.
6. Lack of exercise, excess weight, and a stressful life-style have been shown in some studies to increase the chances of having a heart attack.
7. Other risk factors include sex, race, and age. Women are less likely to have heart attacks than men, perhaps because of protection from their hormonal system. However, after menopause the risk of heart attack in women begins to approach that of men. Blacks are more likely than whites to have high blood pressure and therefore have a higher risk of heart attacks. In addition, the older the person, the more likely that he or she is going to have serious atherosclerosis.

D. SIGNS OF AN IMPENDING HEART ATTACK AND POSSIBLE CARDIAC ARREST

What is it like when a person develops a heart attack? The signals of a heart attack are usually obvious, but they can vary from person to person. The difference between a heart attack and an episode of angina must be understood. *Angina* is the term used to describe a temporary narrowing of a heart artery. This causes pain for several minutes, but permanent damage to the heart muscle does not occur. If the coronary artery does become completely blocked, the damage is irreversible, and a heart attack (myocardial infarction) has occurred.

Angina Pain

Patients who have a heart attack will often have a history of angina. Angina is described as an uncomfortable pressure sensation, often described as squeezing, located in the center of the chest and radiating to the left arm, right arm, up into the neck or jaw, or even into the back. The pain is almost never described as sharp or stabbing. A patient with angina may experience some mild sweating, dizziness, or nausea. Should the pain continue for more than 10 minutes after the patient rests by sitting or lying down, it is likely that a heart attack has occurred.

Heart Attack Pain

The pain of a heart attack, in contrast, feels more severe than that of angina. With a heart attack there is usually profuse sweating, obvious pain, distress, and anxiety. Nausea and vomiting commonly occur. The patient may feel dizzy and short of breath. A sense of impending doom may sweep over the patient, and they may appear irrational.

Many patients who have sudden cardiac arrest will have experienced symptoms of a heart attack prior to their collapse. Remember, however, that often patients will not have experienced symptoms of a heart attack prior to their collapse. Even though they may have underlying heart disease as the cause of their cardiac arrest, they may have nothing more than a brief sense of lightheadedness and then suddenly collapse.

E. "BEAT THE CLOCK"

Once the heart goes into a rhythm that fails to pump blood, the patient will collapse within seconds. Studies have been conducted of patients who had their cardiac rhythm continuously monitored, and then happen to collapse in cardiac arrest. The electrical tracing from the heart revealed that the patients were briefly in a rhythm called ventricular tachycardia, usually for less than a minute. Next they go into ventricular fibrillation. Without CPR a patient will stay in ventricular fibrillation for at most 4 to 5 minutes. With good CPR the ventricular fibrillation will last a little longer, perhaps 10 to 12 minutes. Soon, however, the rhythm of ventricular fibrillation rapidly fades away to a flat line. This absence of electrical activity is called *asystole,* and it announces that the heart is, for all practical purposes, dead. The chances for any treatment approach—drugs, intubation, and open-chest cardiac massage—to resuscitate a heart in asystole are virtually zero.

This means that the rescuers who bring the defibrillator to the patient must literally play "beat the clock" (see Figure 2-1). They must get to a patient in ventricular fibrillation before that remaining electrical activity fades away into asystole. As this book will emphasize, seconds

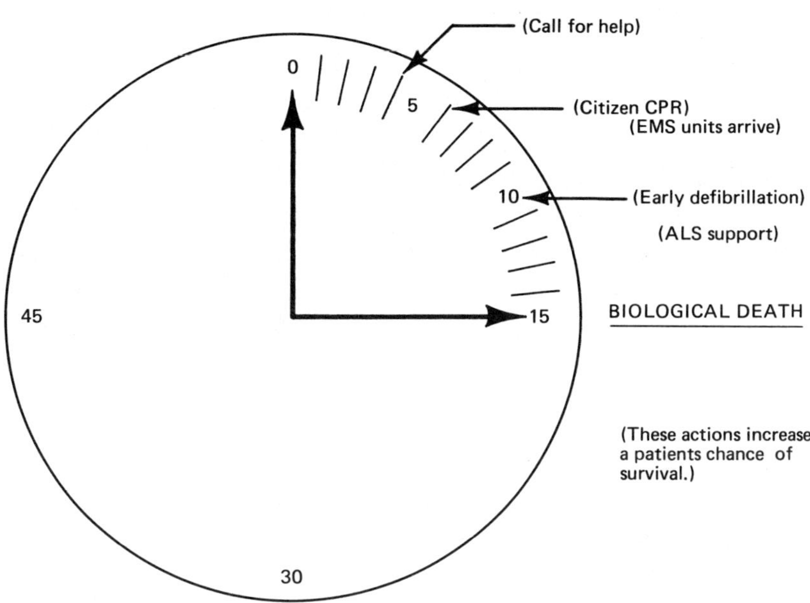

Figure 2–1 "Beat-the-clock" diagram: collapse to call; response time; time to CPR; time to defibrillation.

must be saved in every way possible. The time from a patient's collapse to delivery of the first shock must be as short as possible or the chance of resuscitation will be lost. Automated external defibrillators offer several features that help emergency personnel defibrillate a patient's heart faster.

Chapter 3

RAPID DEFIBRILLATION BY EMTS AND FIRST RESPONDERS

A. WHAT IS DEFIBRILLATION AND A DEFIBRILLATOR?

Defibrillation is the delivery of an electric current directly through the chest wall and heart for the purpose of terminating the deadly rhythm of ventricular fibrillation. In ventricular fibrillation, the electrical system within the heart muscle is chaotically firing hundreds of signals per minute, resulting in no mechanical heartbeat (see Figures 3–1 and 3–2). Delivery of a large jolt of electricity through the heart paralyzes all the muscle cells and wipes out the chaotic signals. If the natural pacemakers of the heart are still viable, they will resume firing in an orderly fashion and their discharges will allow the heart to begin to beat again. The direct-current automatic external defibrillators used for prehospital care contain batteries to store power and a capacitor that can be charged to a high voltage level (see Figure 3–3). This high voltage is then delivered over an extremely brief period of a few milliseconds. It is this high current that paralyzes the cardiac muscle cells.

B. WHAT ROLE DOES CPR PLAY IN EARLY DEFIBRILLATION?

CPR slows the process of dying—it does not sustain life and cannot, by itself, resuscitate a patient in cardiac arrest. What it does do, however, is prolong ventricular fibrillation, and also makes ventricular fibrillation

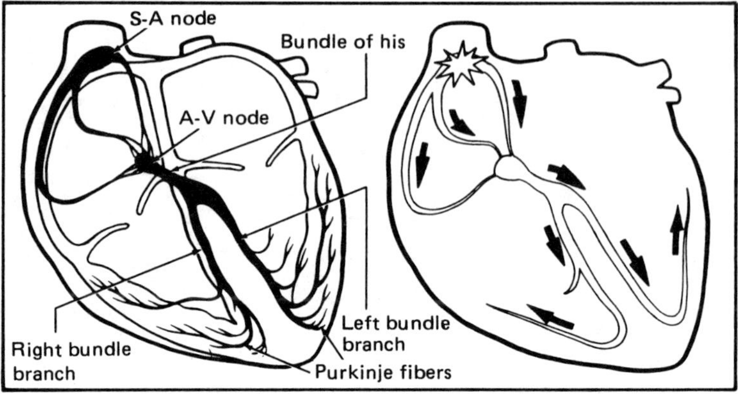

Figure 3–1 Electrical conduction system of the heart. (From Kenneth Stults, *EMT-D Prehospital Defibrillation,* © 1986, p. 21. Reprinted by permission of Prentice-Hall, Inc., Englewood Cliffs, NJ.)

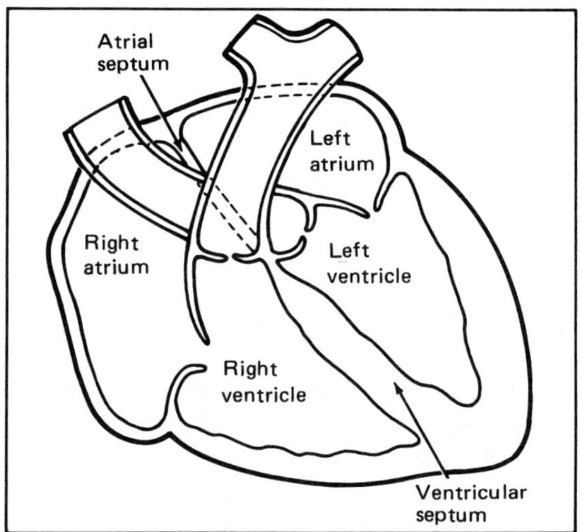

Figure 3–2 Anatomy of the heart. (From Kenneth Stults, *EMT-D Prehospital Defibrillation,* © 1986, p. 17. Reprinted by permission of Prentice-Hall, Inc., Englewood Cliffs, NJ.)

easier to convert once a defibrillatory shock is delivered. The most important effects for CPR occur before the arrival of the rescuer with a defibrillator. This requires that frequent citizen CPR must occur. Bystander CPR increases the likelihood that the rhythm will still be ventricular fibrillation when the defibrillator arrives. Frequent citizen CPR is one of the key ingredients for a successful rapid defibrillation program.

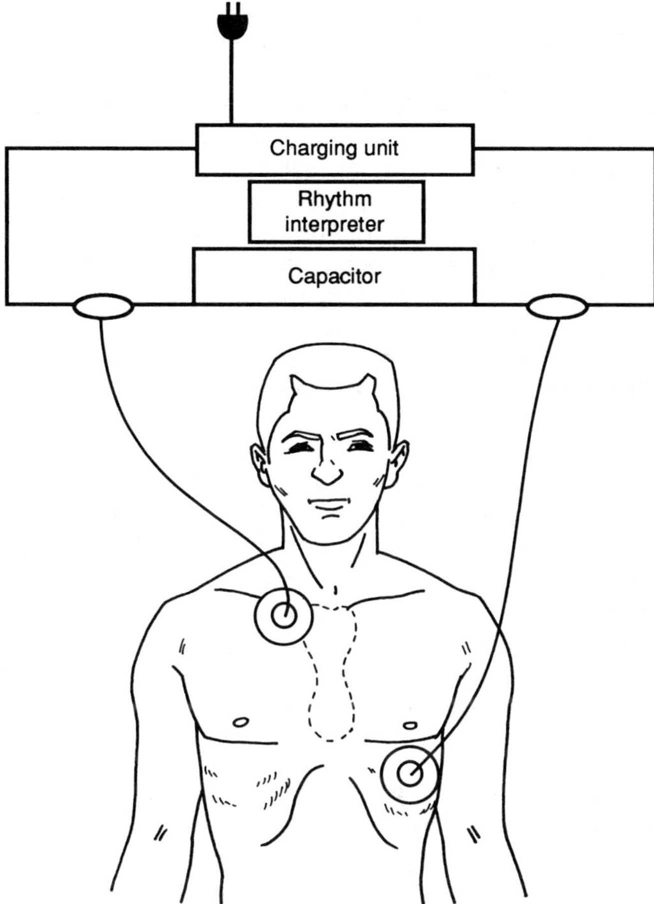

Figure 3–3 Schematic drawing of an AED.

C. MANUAL DEFIBRILLATION: A PROVEN CONCEPT

The first published controlled study of EMT defibrillation appeared in a 1980 issue of the *New England Journal of Medicine*. Numerous additional studies of EMT defibrillation (EMT-D) and first-responder defibrillation have been published in major journals. The Advanced Coronary Treatment (ACT) Foundation and the American College of Emergency Physicians have issued public endorsement of the concept. The American Heart Association at its 1985 National Conference on Standards and Guidelines for Emergency Cardiac Care discussed early defibrillation by

EMTs and first responders and recommended enthusiastically that the concept be implemented.

Early defibrillation is a proven concept—studies from suburban, rural, and urban settings, with and without paramedic backup, have all confirmed that emergency personnel at the EMT and first-responder level can be trained to recognize cardiac rhythms and appropriately operate sophisticated resuscitation equipment. At its core, the success of EMT-D programs is confirmation of the principle of early defibrillation. EMTs and first responders providing early defibrillation will improve survival from our epidemic of sudden cardiac death.

D. EARLY AUTOMATED DEFIBRILLATION: PROVEN EFFECTIVE

The gradual acceptance of EMT-D programs has coincided with the arrival of portable, automatic external defibrillators. These devices have the potential to overcome some of the barriers to the spread of rapid defibrillation programs, such as prolonged and expensive training, poor skill retention, and the need for close medical control. Several field evaluations of these devices have taken place, and controlled trials have helped define the exact place of automated external defibrillators in the care of out-of-hospital sudden cardiac death.

E. ADVANTAGES AND DISADVANTAGES OF THE TWO TYPES OF EARLY DEFIBRILLATION

The advantages and disadvantages of automated versus standard manual defibrillators are highlighted by drawing one distinction: a person interprets the cardiac rhythm with manual defibrillators, whereas a machine interprets the rhythm with automated defibrillators. This distinction introduces several points for an EMT-D or first-responder defibrillation program to consider before making the choice between manual and automatic defibrillators. When all points are considered, we think the clear choice is automated defibrillators for early defibrillation programs.

Initial Training: Rhythm Recognition

In a manual program it takes time to teach EMTs to recognize cardiac rhythms. In a program that uses automated defibrillators, little if any time is needed to teach rhythm recognition. Training can be done without visual displays of rhythms.

Initial Training: Operation of the Device

Automated defibrillators require attachment of adhesive electrode pads to the patient's chest (see Figure 3–4). Through these pads the rhythm is recorded, analyzed, and the electrical shocks are delivered. Because an automatic defibrillator internally recognizes the rhythm, it is programmed to charge the capacitors and, depending on the particular device used, to deliver a shock with little additional action from the operator.

Use of a manual defibrillator is much more complicated and requires many more operator steps, all of which must occur in exact sequence. In general, manual training programs have required 12 hours of initial training; automatic training programs require 2 to 4 hours.

Initial Training: Treatment Protocols

The treatment protocols of the manual defibrillators are presented in detail in a book by Kenneth R. Stults, *EMT-D: Prehospital Defibrillation* (Englewood Cliffs, NJ: Prentice Hall, 1986). The treatment options avail-

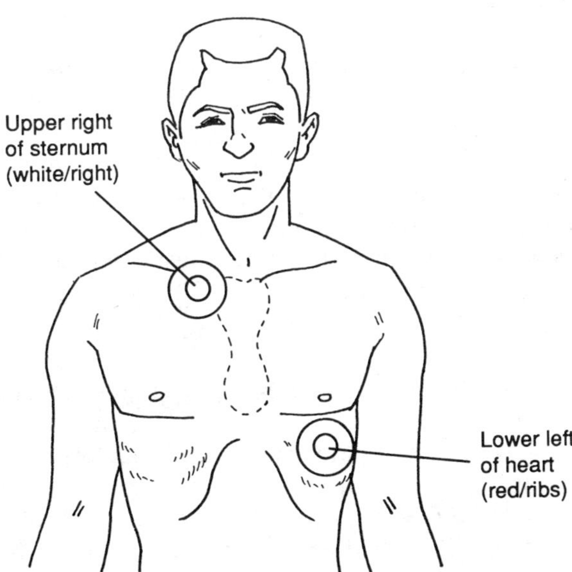

Figure 3–4 Placement of defibrillator pads on a patient's chest. The defibrillator pads are positioned on the anterior chest wall, one to the right of the sternum at the level of the angle of Louis and the second over the apex of the heart.

able to rescuers using automated defibrillators are more limited, and consequently the treatment protocols are simpler and easier to learn and to use.

Maintenance of Skills

Different state EMS systems have adopted different requirements for maintenance of skills. The standards recommended by the National Council of State EMS Training Coordinators state that continued proficiency could be maintained by review sessions that occur from every month to every three months. Automated defibrillators, by not requiring rhythm recognition, have simpler, though not necessarily less frequent, continuing-education classes.

Field Performance: Detection of Ventricular Fibrillation

Inside an automated external defibrillator is electrical circuitry to analyze the rhythm for the presence of ventricular fibrillation. This electrical circuitry for the detection of ventricular fibrillation has been extensively field tested and is under constant refinement. Although automated defibrillators have not been 100 percent accurate in detection of ventricular fibrillation, clinical trials have demonstrated that they do as well as EMTs who use a manual defibrillator. The automated defibrillators occasionally fail to identify and shock extremely fine ventricular fibrillation, and have some trouble with very coarse ventricular fibrillation. So far there have been no reported events where an automated defibrillator delivered a shock to a nonventricular fibrillation rhythm. Automatic defibrillators, on the other hand, are relatively constant in performance. Clinical trials have established that this performance level is completely satisfactory and fully comparable to manual defibrillators.

Field Performance: Nonventricular Fibrillation Detection

The currently available automated defibrillators have, so far, responded appropriately to normal rhythms, or at least rhythms that should not be shocked. EMTs operating manual defibrillators have not done so well. Depending on the program, EMTs can be instructed to be "aggressive" in their approach to rhythms that might be ventricular fibrillation. This means that they occasionally shock rhythms which are asystole or slow, idioventricular rhythms. These acts have not had important clinical consequences, and have remained acceptable in programs that have close medical control.

Speed of Operation

Because of their ease of attachment and operation, and their speed of decision making, automatic external defibrillators are clearly faster than manual defibrillators. Some programs have reported that rescuers can deliver a countershock with an automatic defibrillator an average of 60 seconds faster than they can with a manual defibrillator. This should make an important clinical difference, although such a difference has not yet been observed in clinical studies.

Defibrillation Ability

Technically, "defibrillation" means the removal of ventricular fibrillation. It does not mean conversion of ventricular fibrillation to normal sinus or other perfusing rhythms. The electrical energy delivered by automatic defibrillators, even through their adhesive electrodes, has proven to be as effective at defibrillation as the electrical energy delivered through the paddles of manual defibrillators.

Need for Documentation and Case-by-Case Medical Review

The key to the success of an EMT or first-responder defibrillation program is accurate documentation and close medical review of each case in which a defibrillator is used. This requirement is the same whether an automated or a manual defibrillator is used. **There must be no misunderstanding: Use of an automated defibrillator does not remove the need for medical supervision, and case-by-case review, by a medical doctor or designated program coordinator.**

F. COMMUNITY RESPONDERS

Early defibrillation is now generally accepted as the most effective intervention for cardiac arrest. This means that automatic external defibrillation will inevitably be extended to *community* responders such as policemen, volunteer firefighters, security, and other personnel in corporate settings, airline flight attendants, and staff members of senior centers, nursing homes, and exercise programs. These people have not had the formal 40-hour Department of Transportation first-responder course.

The issues of medical control raised by such possibilities require close attention and are being sorted out by gradual introduction of the devices into such settings. Clinical studies have begun to determine whether or not community responders can be adequately trained to use an automated defibrillator, whether they can retain these skills for long periods, and whether they will correctly operate the device when a cardiac arrest does occur. Early evidence from these studies shows that citizens can indeed learn the following sequence of steps, and (in simulations) perform it within 4 minutes:

1. Verify cardiac arrest.
2. Notify EMS system.
3. Retrieve the automatic defibrillator.
4. Perform one cycle of CPR.
5. Attach the automated defibrillator.
6. Activate the assessment function of the device.
7. Deliver an electric countershock.

Chapter 4

AUTOMATED EXTERNAL DEFIBRILLATORS AND HOW THEY WORK

A. HOW AEDs WORK

Automated external defibrillators (AEDs) are a combination of a defibrillator and a detection system that analyzes the cardiac rhythm. The detection system can diagnose only two rhythms: ventricular fibrillation and nonventricular fibrillation. The currently available defibrillators are attached to the patient with two large adhesive electrodes (Figure 3–4) and connecting cables. The electrical signal from the patient's heart is picked up by the adhesive electrodes and analyzed in the internal circuitry of the automated defibrillator. If the rhythm is ventricular fibrillation (see below for how the AED decides this), a signal is sent to the capacitor to begin to charge. When the capacitors reach their full charge, a shock is delivered through the two adhesive electrodes. The physical characteristics, including energy levels, of the countershocks are virtually identical to countershocks delivered by manual defibrillators.

B. AUTOMATED RHYTHM ANALYSIS

QRS Detection

Look at the example of ventricular fibrillation in Figure 4–1. This looks quite different from the heart's normal rhythm, *normal sinus rhythm.* The tall spiked area in the center of a normal sinus rhythm is

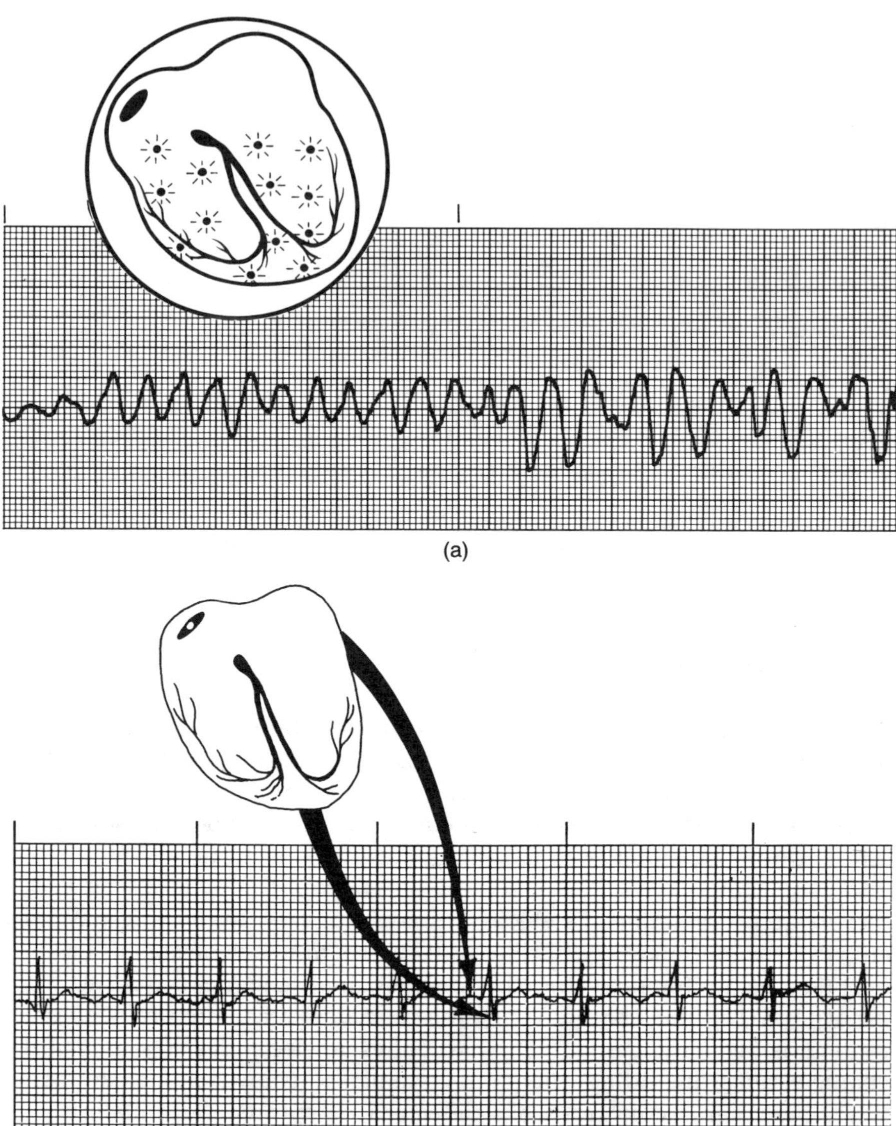

Figure 4–1 Examples of (a) ventricular fibrillation and (b) normal sinus rhythm. (From Kenneth Stults, *EMT-D Prehospital Defibrillation,* © 1986, pp. 50 and 61. Reprinted by permission of Prentice-Hall, Inc., Englewood Cliffs, NJ.)

called the *QRS complex.* Such a pattern never occurs in ventricular fibrillation. One analytic approach that an automatic defibrillator can take is to look for QRS complexes. If they are detected, the automated take is to look for QRS complexes. If they are detected, the automated defibrillator will decide that ventricular fibrillation is not present. This is a safety check that automated defibrillators always use.

Ventricular Fibrillation Frequency

You can see that ventricular fibrillation looks like a lot of up-and-down squiggles. These squiggles are actually an electrical summation of innumerable areas of electrical activity in the heart. From the top of one squiggle to the top of the next is referred to as a *cycle of ventricular fibrillation.* You can describe a particular example of ventricular fibrillation in terms of how many of these cycles occur per second (a unit of measure called *hertz*) or how many occur per minute (the easiest to measure visually). Most cases of ventricular fibrillation have a frequency of 150 to 300 cycles per minute.

Ventricular Fibrillation Amplitude

You can also see that the squiggles go up and down to different degrees. This is called the *amplitude* or height of the signal. An electrical signal of 1 millivolt from the patient will make a deflection on the monitor screen of 1 centimeter. One brand of semiautomatic defibrillator has a one-dimensional monitor light that also moves 1 centimeter in response to 1 millivolt of electrical energy from the patient. There is no firm point at which the electrical activity of ventricular fibrillation fades away and becomes asystole. In general, when the electrical signal has an amplitude of less than 1 millimeter on the ECG paper, it is no longer considered to be ventricular fibrillation but is referred to as asystole.

C. PUTTING IT TOGETHER

In the simplest terms, the rhythm analysis system of automated defibrillators looks at all of these features: the absence of anything that looks like a QRS complex, the frequency of the signal, the amplitude of the signal, and a special integration of frequency and amplitude called *slope* (see Figure 4–2). The rhythm analysis system "takes a look" at the rhythm coming from the patient for brief periods of time – usually 2 to 3 seconds. If it sees a rhythm that meets the characteristics of ventricular fibrillation – and usually this means no QRS complexes, a frequency greater than 150 cycles per minute, and an amplitude greater than 1 to 3 millimeters – the automated defibrillator begins to get excited. Depending on the manufacturer, the device will recheck the rhythm several more times. If these checks confirm the presence of ventricular fibrilla-

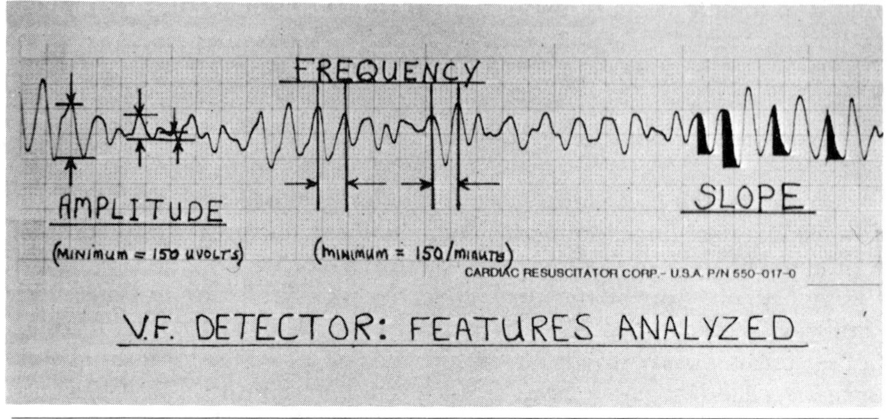

Figure 4–2 Features of the cardiac rhythm analyzed by AED.

tion, the fully automatic defibrillator begins to charge its capacitor, while checking the rhythm one more time. If this final check still indicates ventricular fibrillation, the device will deliver the countershock.

Semiautomated defibrillators, after confirming ventricular fibrillation, do not automatically charge their capacitors and deliver a shock. Instead, they give a message to the operator that a shock is "advised," and the operator must then push the shock button. Once the shock button is pushed, the capacitor begins to charge (in one device, the capacitors begin to charge as soon as the "analyze" button is pushed), and when fully charged the shock is delivered. When the charge is delivered to a human body, there is a sudden jerking movement as the electrical current suddenly causes all the muscles to contract.

D. THE PROBLEM OF STOPPING CPR

There must be no contact with the patient while the AEDs analyze the rhythm, charge the capacitors, and deliver the countershocks. This means that the rescuer must stop chest compressions, ventilation efforts, and not touch the patient in any way. This is to permit accurate analysis of the cardiac rhythm and to prevent accidental shocks to the rescuer. In addition, the movements of CPR can cause the automated defibrillators to stop their analysis process. How long must CPR stop? With the automatic defibrillator the time between stopping CPR (activating the rhythm analyzer) and the delivery of a countershock will be between 10 and 15 seconds. With the semiautomated defibrillators this period will be between 15 and 25 seconds.

Can CPR be safely stopped for such long periods? The American Heart Association recommends that CPR not be stopped for longer than 5 seconds. Use of an automated defibrillator requires that CPR be stopped for at least 10 to 15 seconds, often more. The dilemma is one of a trade-off between the negative effects of stopping CPR and the positive effects of delivering a defibrillatory shock.

It must be restated in no uncertain terms: **CPR cannot return a spontaneously perfusing rhythm to a heart in ventricular fibrillation, but defibrillation can.** The answer is clear—the potential benefit of the electrical shocks far outweighs the negative effects of a brief delay in CPR. The 1986 Standards and Guidelines for Cardiac Arrest and Emergency Cardiac Care of the American Heart Association recognize this and state that when using automated external defibrillators, CPR can be stopped for up to 15 seconds. In fact, in the treatment protocols, for patients who remain in ventricular fibrillation after the first electrical countershock, CPR may be interrupted for even longer periods—up to 1 minute. Again, the potential value of two or three countershocks in this period justifies interrupting CPR.

Chapter 5

MEDICAL DIRECTION AND PROGRAM QUALITY

A. THE CONCEPT OF MEDICAL CONTROL

An EMT or first responder who performs a medical procedure (other than transportation) in an emergency engages in the practice of medicine. Over the past decade, prehospital care personnel have been permitted by law to perform more and more medical procedures in their efforts to save people from death and disability. In many parts of the country EMT-As and first responders operate independently of physician contact, and medical review of the patient's treatment seldom, if ever, occurs. This situation arose most often when programs were started in communities where no physicians were available, interested, or qualified to offer assistance. Lack of medical leadership has frequently limited the contribution of EMTs and first responders.

In many locations basic life support squads maintain only a nominal medical control relationship with a physician. The topic of medical control for basic life support care is a vigorously debated subject today and many possible changes are possible over the next several years. Medical control would assure high-quality performance in emergency care by providing physician review of emergency personnel performance and physician assistance in patient management. Medical control also provides legal protection for the EMS rescuers in many situations by shifting responsibility to a physician.

B. MEDICAL CONTROL FOR EARLY DEFIBRILLATION PROGRAMS

Every defibrillation program for EMTs and first responders *must* have formal medical control. Although the details required by emergency medical service programs may differ from state to state, this formal medical control must be established by these features:

1. *Medical director.* A designated physician must understand and accept the responsibility of being the medical director of an early defibrillation program.
2. *Training program.* A physician must approve the content and the presentation of the training program. The physician, or a representative, should provide the instruction (see Appendix V for a detailed outline of a training curriculum).
3. *Standing orders.* The medical director must approve the standing orders that will be used by the emergency personnel.
4. *Certification.* The medical director must approve the certification process: the methods used to test the students, including written examinations and demonstrations of practical skills.
5. *Authorization.* After certification, the medical director must issue formal "authorization" to operate the defibrillator according to the standing orders.
6. *Case-by-case review.* In every event in which defibrillators are used (or potentially should have been used) the emergency situation must be reviewed by the medical director or designated representative. This involves medical review of every incident in which cardiopulmonary resuscitation is performed. These so-called "CPR cases" are not limited to cardiac arrest due to heart disease, but include drownings, traumatic arrest, drug overdoses, and respiratory failure. There are two ways in which case-by-case review occurs: by a written report and by review of the recordings made by the voice/electrocardiographic tape recorders attached to automated defibrillators.

REQUIREMENTS
FOR MEDICAL CONTROL

1. Medical director
2. Training program
3. Standing orders
4. Certification
5. Authorization
6. Case-by-case review

C. THE CONCEPT OF STANDING ORDERS

The medical director issues operating instructions for the automated defibrillators in the form of standing orders. Early defibrillation programs have found standing orders for cardiac arrest resuscitations to be extremely effective and successful.

The concept that physicians have *direct* control over the decision making in the field by EMTs and first responders is an understandable one but is impractical and accompanied by many problems. Because quickness is so important during a cardiac arrest, nothing should get in the way of rapid delivery of a defibrillatory shock. Radio contact and telemetric transmission of an electrocardiographic recording to a base station physician presents many potential delays and is considered inappropriate for early defibrillation programs. To our knowledge all early defibrillation programs currently in service in the United States use the standing-order approach. Figure 5–1 presents the American Heart Association treatment sequence for ventricular fibrillation modified for emergency medical technicians trained to defribrillate and first responders.

Standing orders, in effect, are a direct order from the program medical director to perform certain tasks for a patient. The emergency rescuer must always operate under the authority of the medical director's medical license. When the rescuer completes the AED training course successfully, he or she receives a certificate of authorization. The certificate is, in effect, a "prescription" from the medical director that legally authorizes the first responder to use the AED *in certain situations and in a prescribed manner.* Standing orders present exactly what these "certain situations" and "certain manners" are. Appendix II presents an example of the type of standing orders, or authorization certificate, that must be issued to emergency personnel. Note the additional details in the appendices regarding the standing orders. These details provide exact performance guidelines.

D. WRITTEN DOCUMENTATION BY RESCUERS

An EMS incident report is an important medical document (see Figure 5–2). It should follow the SOAP format and should be complete. During a cardiac arrest many events occur and the incident report provides an opportunity to supply additional explanatory details. For example, patient care may have been delayed because of the location of the cardiac arrest, such as a small bathroom or the scene of a motor vehicle accident.

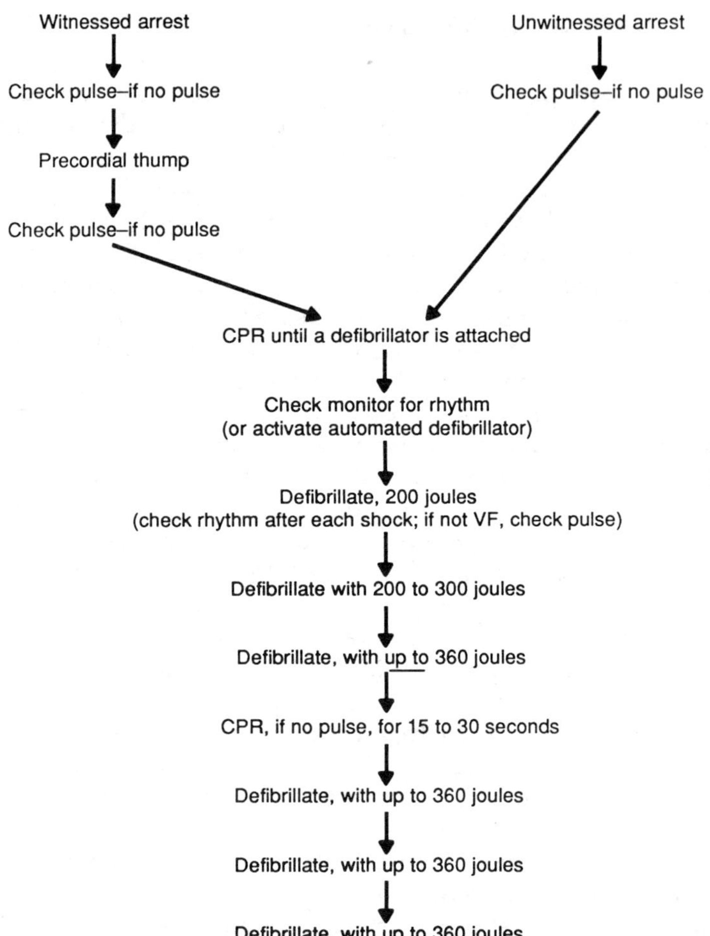

Figure 5-1 American Heart Association treatment sequence for ventricular fibrillation. The chart has been modified for EMT-D and first defibrillation programs. [Adapted with permission from "Standards and Guidelines for Cardiopulmonary Resuscitation (CPR) and Emergency Cardiac Care (ECC)." JAMA 255:2905, 1986.]

E. VERBAL DOCUMENTATION BY RESCUERS

The voice/ECG recording begins whenever the automated defibrillator is turned on, either when the lid is lifted or when the operator presses the power switch. A continuous running commentary by the defibrillator operator should begin. The emergency care provider should describe all

Blood Run No.

Agency Incident No.

KING COUNTY
EMERGENCY MEDICAL SERVICES
INCIDENT REPORT

Mo	Day	Yr	
0 9	1 5	8 3	07142

Agency Name: UNIVERSITY F.D. — No. 9 8

Are You First EMS Reporting Agency On Scene? 1 ☑ YES 2 ☐ NO

Incident Site & City: 4052 ESSEX AVE N.

Responding In F.D.: 9 8

Patient Name: FRANK BOMAN

SEX: 1 ☑ M 2 ☐ F — Age: Yr. 6 2 Mo. — Pt#: 1/1 — AID UNIT No. 2 0 — MEDIC UNIT No. 5 2 — Geo Code 02

Patient Address: 4052 ESSEX AVE N. — City & State: SEATTLE, WASH. — Phone: 555-3686

Nearest Relative Name: EDITH BOMAN — Relation: WIFE — Phone

Private Physician Name: ROBERT KING — Hospital or Clinic: UNIVERSITY HOSPITAL — Phone

ACTION TAKEN

1 ☐ Examine Only
3 ☐ No Exam (Unneeded)
2 ☑ Examine & Assist
4 ☐ Exam/Treatment Refused

INCIDENT CODE

Mechanism: M D
Type: 2 1 8

SEVERITY

1 ☐ Non urgent
3 ☑ Immediate Life Threat
2 ☐ Urgent
4 ☐ Not Applicable

PROCEDURES

1 ☑ O_2
2 ☐ Wound Care
3 ☐ Extrication/Rescue
4 ☐ Splinting
5 ☑ Oral Airway/Bag Mask
6 ☑ ECG Monitor
7 ☐ Esophageal Obturator
8 ☑ CPR
9 ☐ Plan A - 1
10 ☐ Plan A - 2
11 ☐ Plan B
12 ☐ Endotracheal Intubation
13 ☐ IV - Central Line
14 ☐ IV - Peripheral
15 ☑ Manual DC Shock by an EMT
16 ☐ Intracardiac Injection
17 ☐ Flutter Valve
18 ☐ Pericardiocentesis
19 ☐ Cricothyrotomy
20 ☐ Shock Trouser
21 ☐ Automatic DC Shock by an EMT
Other ______

PROCED NUMBER 12 - 21 ONLY	EMS NUMBER
1 5	0 0 1

ECG RHYTHM

1 ☐ Sinus
2 ☐ V Fib
3 ☐ V Tach
4 ☐ Asystole
5 ☐ Idioventricular
6 ☐ Other
7 ☐ Unknown

DR. CONTACTED 1 ☑ YES 2 ☐ NO

Name of Doctor and Hospital Contacted:
1. MEDIC #512 DR. LERCH UNIVERSITY HOSPITAL
2. ______

CPR

CPR INITIATED BY
1 ☑ Fire Department
2 ☑ Paramedic
3 ☐ Ambulance
4 ☐ MD/RN
5 ☐ Citizen with Dispatcher Assistance
6 ☐ Citizen without Dispatcher Assistance

NAME OF CITIZEN INITIATING CPR: JANET HELMS
Phone: 555-3771

WAS CITIZEN PREVIOUSLY TRAINED? 1 ☐ Yes 2 ☐ No 3 ☐ Unknown

LOCATION OF CARDIAC ARREST
1 ☑ Home
2 ☐ Residence other than home
3 ☐ Work
4 ☐ Public place
5 ☐ Nursing home
6 ☐ Other

WAS CARDIAC ARREST WITNESSED? 1 ☑ Yes 2 ☐ No 3 ☐ Unknown

WAS DISPATCHER-ASSISTED CPR OFFERED? 1 ☑ Yes 2 ☐ No 3 ☐ Unknown

ESTIMATED TIME FROM COLLAPSE TO: (Min.)
Agency Call: 0 1
Initiation Of CPR: 0 4
Definitive Care: 1 0

OUTCOME
1 ☐ Expired At Scene/ER
2 ☑ Admit To ICU/CCU
3 ☐ Unknown

Time Of Call (24 Hr.): 1 9 4 1

Response Time (Min.): AID 0 4 — MEDIC 1 0

Out Of Service Time (Min.): AID — MEDIC

Source Of Alarm:
1 ☑ Citizen
2 ☐ Police
3 ☐ MD/RN
4 ☐ F.D.
5 ☐ Ambulance
6 ☐ Other

Responding From Quarters? 1 ☑ Yes 1 ☐ No

Transported To: UNIV. HOSP. 2 9

Transported By: MEDIC 512 5 2

Ambulance Response Time (Min.)

FOR AGENCY USE:

PERSONNEL AID	PARAMEDIC	EMS NUMBER
1 JOHN LUPTON, EMT-D	1	
2 KATHY PETERSON	2	
3 JOE RAMIREZ	3	

SIGNATURE OF PERSON COMPLETING REPORT: John Lupton

Figure 5–2 Example of written incident report. (Adapted from M.K. Copass, ed., et al., *EMT Defibrillation,* Emergency Training, Westport, CT, © EDI 1984.)

	POSITION	BLOOD PRESSURE	PULSE RATE	RESPIRATORY RATE	CONSCIOUSNESS	PUPILS
VITAL SIGNS	⟷	0 /	0	0 / Min. Est. Air Exchange ☐ Normal ☐ Increased ☐ Decreased	☐ Alert ☐ Semi-Conscious ☑ Comatose	☐ Conjugate ☐ Dysconjugate ☐ Reactive ☑ Unreactive ☑ Dilated ☐ Mid ☐ Constricted
	↳	/				
TIME	↕	/				

FLOW CHART TIME →	1946	1959	2001	2002									
Blood Pressure	0	144/92	140/94	126/94									
Pulse Rate	0	110	120	120									
Respiratory Rate	0	8/M	8/M	8/M									
Consciousness	COM	COM	COM	COM									
Pupils	F&D	M=R	M=R	M=R									
Rhythm (ECG)	VF	3° BLK	3° BLK	—									
Morphine													
Oxygen	11 LT	11 LT	11 LT	11 LT									
DC Shock (400 JOULES)	YES												

Medications Taken By Patient At Home

Narrative (Subjective, Objective, Assessment, Plan) S. A 62 YR OLD ♂ CARDIAC ARREST. PTS WIFE STATED THAT HER HUSBAND HAD BEEN HAVING SOME CHEST PAIN EARLIER TODAY AND HAD JUST STOPPED BREATHING SHORTLY BEFORE OUR ARRIVAL. SHE ALSO STATED THAT PT. HAD JUST COME OUT OF THE HOSPITAL LAST FRIDAY. PMH_x: MEDICAL — ANGINA, CHF — MEDS: UNKNOWN

O. UPON ARRIVAL PT. WAS SUPINE ON LIVING ROOM FLOOR — UNCONSCIOUS, UNRESPONSIVE, NO PULSE, NO RESP., AND CYANOTIC IN COLOR, NO LIFE SIGNS. C.P.R. WAS NOT IN PROGRESS UPON ARRIVAL BUT WAS ATTEMPTED BY WIFE PRIOR TO OUR ARRIVAL. HEENT — PUP FIX AND DILATED, NECK VEINS DISTENT, PT CYANOTIC, ECG — VENT-FIB

ASS. CARDIAC ARR.

PLAN — C.P.R. INITIATED UPON ARRIVAL - HEART MONITOR HOOK-UP - 1 COUNTERSHOCK ADMIN. PRIOR TO MEDIC 512 ARRIVAL — STRIP IS ATTACHED - BAG MASK WITH 100% O_2 @ 11 LITERS. BASIC LIFE SUPPORT ADMIN. APPROX 6 MIN BEFORE PT LIFE SIGNS CAME BACK. MEDIC 512 ALSO ADMIN I.V. & LIDOCAINE, ATROPINE @ APPROX 1956 HOURS TRANS TO U.H. VIA MEDIC 512 WITH REQUIRED BAG MASK ASSIST ONLY.

AGENCY COPY

FORM 911 1/83

Figure 5-2 (continued)

the steps of the standing orders as he or she carries them out. The following should be included:

1. *Brief introduction.* "Hello, doctor, this is EMT Steve Marth on the scene of a presumed cardiac arrest. The patient is a 57-year-old male, and CPR is being performed by my partner."
2. *Description of the attachment of the automated defibrillator.* "I am now attaching the defib pads to the patient, one to the right sternum and one to the left lower ribs."
3. *Description of the treatment cycles.* "I am now going to automatic mode. Everybody stand clear! One-one thousand, two-one thousand, three-one thousand. . . . It appeared that one shock was delivered."
4. *Description of the CPR cycles.* "Switching from automatic mode and going back to CPR for 15 seconds. One-one thousand, two-one thousand. . . . Checking now for a pulse. There does appear to be a pulse!"
5. *Description of other care.* "We are now checking the blood pressure, which is 100 over 60. The patient is beginning to make efforts to breathe. We have stopped chest compressions and will support the patient with oxygen via a bag valve mask."

RESPONSIBILITIES OF EMT-Ds AND FIRST RESPONDERS

1. Proper and current certification
2. Maintenance of skills
3. Performance according to standing orders
4. Proper equipment maintenance
5. Proper control of scene—**safety!**
6. Written and verbal documentation of events
7. Postevent case-by-case review

F. REVIEW OF VOICE/ECG TAPE RECORDINGS

The key to providing close medical control is dual-channel tape recorders attached to portable defibrillators. These allow electronic reconstruction (and legal documentation) of each cardiac arrest. In these devices, a standard or mini-tape cassette records not only the electrocardiographic tracing from the patient but also the verbal reports provided by the rescuers at the scene. An incident report and the cassette tape from the defibrillator must be sent to the program coordinator or the medical director within 24 hours of the incident.

All AEDs discussed in this book use ferrous oxide audio recording tape, and demodulators or transcribers can be purchased from the manufacturers. The demodulator or transcriber for the cassette tape is used to play back the rhythm of the patient, and the verbal report of the first responder. The program coordinator reads the incident report, listens to the verbal account from the scene, and reviews the recorded rhythm to identify whether the performance by the rescuers and the automated defibrillator was correct:

1. Did the rescuers quickly and efficiently attach the defibrillator while maintaining effective CPR?
2. Did the rescuers obtain a clear rhythm tracing for the AED to interpret?
3. Was the assessment of the presence or absence of ventricular fibrillation by the AED correct?
4. Did the AED make the right decision to deliver or not to deliver a countershock?
5. Was the AED operated correctly and safely?
6. Were other aspects of patient care satisfactory?

If necessary to understand all the events, the coordinator calls the individual emergency personnel and reviews the field treatment in detail. Cardiac arrests in which an electric countershock was delivered, as well as any potential problem cases, are reviewed with the medical director.

G. INNOVATIVE APPROACHES TO EVENT DOCUMENTATION

Several innovative approaches to the tasks of event documentation, record keeping, and data management have been developed and incorporated into automated defibrillators. These include solid-state memory modules and magnetic tape that store a variety of information with each clinical use of the device. These include segments of the rhythm tracing and notations on the operations of the defibrillator. Special playback units connected to computers and printers can provide an instant hard copy for medical control review (Figure 5–3).

HEARTSTART 2000		RUN REPORT	
REPORT DATE ____/____/____		TECHNICIANS ________________	
		________________	
EPISODE DATE	20 FEB 87	PART NUMBER	900050
EPISODE TIME	08:18:34	SERIAL NUMBER	000421
SELF CHECK	OK	SOFTWARE VERSION	9
CONFIGURATION	SEMI-AUTO	MCU S.W. VERSION	4

EVENT LOG:

______	DATE: 20 FEB 87 ______
08:18:34	UNIT ON
08:18:43	"CHECK PATIENT" MESSAGE GIVEN—TREATABLE RHYTHM DETECTED
08:18:46	START ANALYSIS
08:18:50	START CHARGING
08:18:53	COMMIT TO TREAT
08:18:54	READY TO SHOCK
08:18:57	SHOCK NUMBER 1 DELIVERED, 100 JOULES
08:19:04	START ANALYSIS
08:19:08	START CHARGING
08:19:14	COMMIT TO TREAT
08:19:15	READY TO SHOCK
08:19:18	SHOCK NUMBER 2 DELIVERED, 200 JOULES
08:19:24	START ANALYSIS
08:19:31	SHOCK NOT INDICATED
08:20:52	"CHECK PATIENT" MESSAGE GIVEN—TREATABLE RHYTHM DETECTED
08:21:00	START ANALYSIS
08:21:04	START CHARGING
08:21:07	COMMIT TO TREAT
08:21:18	READY TO SHOCK
08:21:27	SHOCK NUMBER 3 DELIVERED, 360 JOULES
08:21:36	START ANALYSIS
08:21:42	SHOCK NOT INDICATED
08:27:55	"CHECK PATIENT" MESSAGE GIVEN—TREATABLE RHYTHM DETECTED
08:27:57	"CHECK ELECTRODES" MESSAGE GIVEN
08:27:57	UNIT OFF

SER. NO. 000421 EPISODE DATE: 20 FEB 87 TIME: 08:18:34

Figure 5–3 Sample printout from a solid-state medical control module. The module displays rhythm segments of ventricular fibrillation, one shock and postshock rhythm, as well as annotations made on run reports. (Courtesy King County EMS Division, Department of Public Health.)

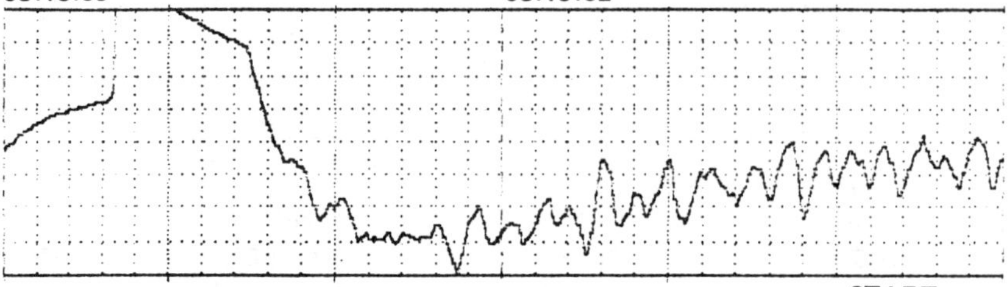

08:18:59
08:19:02
START
ANALYSIS

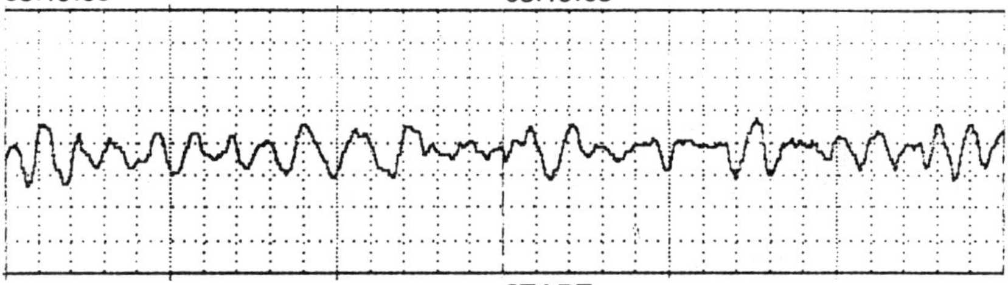

08:19:05
08:19:08
START
CHARGING

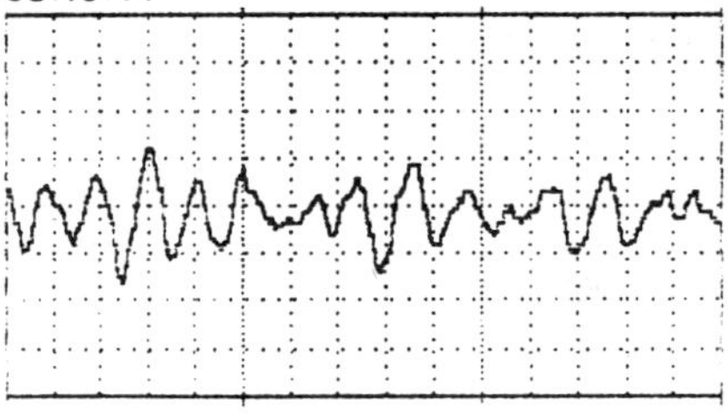

08:19:11

SHOCK NUMBER 2 DATA:
TIME DELIVERED . . . . 08:19:18 BATTERY . . . . . GOOD
ENERGY DELIVERED . . . 200 JOULES IMPEDANCE . . . . . 80 OHMS

08:19:19
08:19:22
START
ANALYSIS

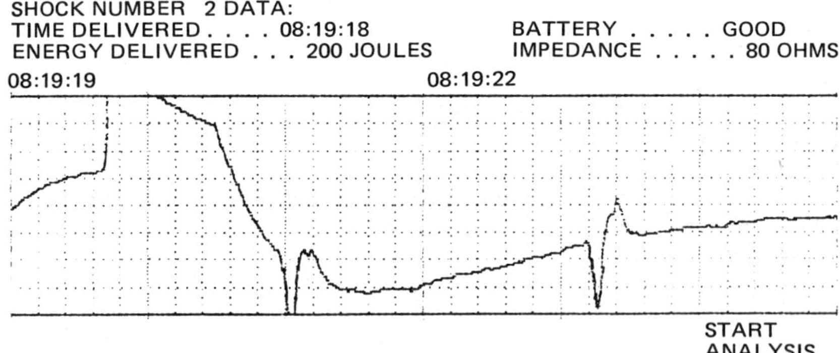

SER. NO. 000421 EPISODE DATE: 20 FEB 87 TIME: 08:18:34

Figure 5–3 (continued)

H. SOLID-STATE MEDICAL CONTROL MODULE VERSUS VOICE/ECG TAPE RECORDINGS

The new approaches to medical control conveniently allow accurate review of the following performance items:

1. Whether the defibrillator was properly attached
2. The number of times the EMTs or first responders assessed the patient's rhythm by pressing ANALYZE
3. The rhythm upon initial device attachment, during each analysis period, immediately after each shock, and for each minute of rhythm monitoring
4. The total number and energy level of shocks delivered
5. If CPR and artifact were absent during the rhythm analysis periods
6. How quickly the personnel performed their tasks

In contrast, tape cassettes with the voice recording and with the capacity to record the rhythm continuously provide information not available on the printouts from the event documentation systems:

1. A sense of the "command of the scene" by the emergency personnel, their air of confidence, the smoothness and efficiency with which they perform their tasks; their overall professionalism
2. Their ability to troubleshoot the scene in terms of numerous unexpected problems that can occur in the field and in terms of interactions with bystanders, family members, and other personnel
3. Their ability to troubleshoot any equipment problems that occur
4. Their attention to the patient, to ventilation, to proper CPR, and to periodic reassessments of the patient's status
5. The proper selection and administration of advanced life support interventions such as intubation and medications (in those systems where the level of the EMTs permitted such interventions)
6. Their attention to safety: to an insistence on no contact with the patient during each rhythm analysis period and during each shock delivery

An example of a program coordinator's review sheet is shown in Figure 5–4.

I. MAINTENANCE OF SKILLS

Depending on the rate of cardiac arrest in the community, an emergency responder may go several years without treating a patient in cardiac

Review method
(–) Magnetic tape
(–) Medical control module

Not Able to Decide	Fail	Satisfactory	Excellent	Skill Areas	Criteria to Pass
(–)	0	1 2 3	4	Communication/ Command of scene	1. Verifies arrest/begins CPR 2. Attaches defibrillator pads Opens semiautomatic external defibrillator and communicates identifying information
(–)	0	1 2 3	4	Defibrillation	1. Stops CPR/clears patient 2. Presses "analyze" to assess 3. If "shock indicated" ascertains patient is cleared and presses "shock" 4. Presses "analyze" to reassess 5. If "shock indicated" ascertains patient is cleared and presses "shock" 6. Presses "analyze" to reassess again 7. If "shock indicated" ascertains patient is cleared and presses "shock" 8. Resumes CPR for 15-60 sec 9. Repeats proper sequence delivering shocks 4, 5, and 6 if persistent ventricular fibrillation
(–)	0	1 2 3	4	Patient support/ Assessment	1. Checks pulse if "no shock indicated" 2. Does CPR on pulseless patients 3. If pulse, takes blood presure: if under 60 palpable, continues CPR 4. If blood pressure over 60 palpable, monitors respirations and ventilations
(–)	0	1 2 3	4	Safety (must pass)	1. Always clears patient prior to "analyze" and "shock"
(–)	0	1 2 3	4	Speed	1. Can hook up, turn on, and make first assessment within 90 sec

Table score (max = 20) (–)

Figure 5–4 Example of a program coordinator's case-by-case event documentation review sheet. (Courtesy King County EMS Division, Department of Public Health.)

arrest. Is she or he going to perform correctly? There are three ways that a program can guarantee proper performance of such a rare event—practice, practice, and practice. How often and in what format should practice occur?

Frequency of Practice

The minimal answer to the question "How often?" is initial training and no formal skill review. This makes the assumption that the details of equipment operation can be remembered for up to several years. The National Council of State EMS Training Coordinators and other organizations involved with early defibrillation programs consider this unacceptable. At the other extreme are monthly drills. The EMT automated defibrillation program in King County, Washington, observed that practice drills at 6-month intervals did not maintain satisfactory skill performance. At the present time most systems permit a maximum of 90 days between practice drills and have found this to be satisfactory. Many emergency personnel choose to drill even more frequently, up to once a month.

Unscheduled and Undocumented Review

The most successful long-term skill maintenance occurs when individual EMTs and first responders voluntarily, on their own initiative, spend a few minutes each shift with a quick check of the equipment. This may involve nothing more than a visual inspection of the AED controls, a mental review of the steps they would follow in the event of a cardiac arrest, and which controls they would operate. If at all possible, the program coordinator and medical director should encourage this attitude of personal and individual review.

Content of Practice Sessions

The practice sessions can be as elaborate as personnel interest and time allow. The following is the recommended *minimum* content of a 1-hour practice session which should occur at least every 90 days:

RECOMMENDED MINIMAL CONTENT OF PRACTICE SESSIONS

1. Take role (for documentation purposes)
2. Performance review of recent patients
3. Equipment review (if needed)
4. Instructor demonstration of standing orders
5. Discussion of rhythm treatment possibilities—scenario-playing
6. Practice of field protocols with manikin and defibrillator
7. Objective skills test (see Figure 5–4)

Chapter 6

SPECIAL SITUATIONS

A. MONITORING THE CONSCIOUS PATIENT WITH CHEST PAIN

The Role of Monitoring

Rescuers will frequently arrive at the side of a person who is having a heart attack but has not gone into cardiac arrest. The person may be having chest pain, shortness of breath, and may be covered in sweat. Even though the patient is conscious and may be talking to the rescuer, the person may collapse into cardiac arrest at any second. Similarly, even patients in mild distress from chest pain have a chance of going into cardiac arrest while they are under the care of the rescuers. In these circumstances the personnel may want to attach the monitor leads of the automatic defibrillator.

Monitoring is most useful when rescuers have been trained to recognize cardiac rhythms. In general, when a defibrillation program has decided to proceed with AEDs, that program accepts the lack of rhythm monitoring by rescuers. Since the decision to deliver defibrillatory shock is given to the automated defibrillator, why should the rescuers be expected to monitor the rhythm of conscious chest pain patients? Nevertheless, even EMTs or first responders who have not had formal rhythm recognition training learn to recognize the chaotic pattern of ventricular fibrillation in a patient whom they are monitoring.

If a monitored patient becomes unresponsive, the rescuers should quickly resume CPR and proceed to attach the defibrillator pads as rapidly as possible. Once the pads are attached the rescuers should follow the operation steps described in Chapter 5.

Never Forget the Patient

Emergency personnel must never be distracted by their equipment to the point that the patient is neglected. This is particularly true when monitoring conscious patients. These patients may have low blood pressure, shortness of breath, agitation, and severe pain. It is not helpful to these patients for the rescuer to spend inappropriate amounts of time attaching the monitor leads and staring at an interesting rhythm. Care of the patient rather than care of the equipment always comes first!

B. TROUBLESHOOTING THE DEFIBRILLATORS

A rescuer must learn to recognize the most common equipment problems that can occur while treating patients in cardiac arrest. Each of these problems should trigger a mental checklist of possible causes and possible solutions. The two most common problems with automated defibrillators are problems with the contact between the skin and the defibrillator pads, and problems with excessive motion of the patient.

Inadequate Contact between the Skin and the Defibrillatory Pads

Automatic and semiautomatic defibrillators send a high-frequency signal between the two adhesive defibrillatory pads. The conductive pathway between these two pads must have low resistance *(impedance)* in order for the signal to travel. Anything that interferes with the passage of this signal between the two defibrillatory pads will be detected by the device, and alarm signals will indicate that the defibrillatory pads are not connected properly. Some automated defibrillators provide a voice recording that states: "Turn off defibrillator. Connect electrodes." A light also flashes next to the message "Loose electrodes" and the monitor and paper strip display a distinctive squared-off signal. Other defibrillators provide written phrases such as "Connect electrodes" or "Check electrodes" on the LCD display screen.

There are many causes for poor contact between the adhesive monitor patches and the patient's skin. Whenever alarm signals are received, the rescuers should immediately go through the following troubleshooting checklist:

1. *Press firmly against the defibrillatory pads* to make sure that the adhesive is stuck to the skin and that the conductive surface of the pad is making contact with the chest. Often, this is the only troubleshooting that is needed.
2. *Quickly recheck all connections* between the defibrillator pads and the cables, and between the cables and the automatic defibrillator.
3. *Hairy chest?* A small safety razor should be carried to shave quickly a small area of the chest beneath the defibrillator pads.
4. *Sweaty or wet chest?* Patients with severe chest pain who have a cardiac arrest are often covered in perspiration. They may also be wet from rain or from immersion. The easiest approach: Use the patient's underclothing or shirt to wipe the chest dry quickly. Also carry alcohol swabs, 4 x 4 gauze, and a small towel to dry the patient's chest.
5. *Small, bony, or irregularly shaped chest?* If necessary, the defibrillatory pads can be moved approximately one-half the pad diameter and repositioned on another area of the chest to see if better contact can be achieved.
6. *Dry, outdated, or defective defibrillatory pads?* If loose electrodes continue to be indicated, the defibrillatory pads should quickly be replaced with another set. **A spare set of pads should always be carried!** In addition, the electrode gel can slowly evaporate from some brands of defibrillator pads. A tube of defibrillator electrode gel should be available so that a small amount of gel can be placed on the nonadhesive or conductive portion of the pads if it appears that the pads may be too dry. Recently, some defibrillator manufacturers have equipped their defibrillator pads with a "conductive adhesive" so that this problem of evaporation of electrode gel should not occur.

Excessive Motion of the Patient

The automatic detection systems cannot properly operate when either the patient or the device are moving. Artifact signals from motion can prevent countershocks from being delivered to patients in ventricular fibrillation. In addition, there is some possibility that motion signals can be misinterpreted as ventricular fibrillation by automatic defibrillators. The possibility exists that the device could charge its capacitors and deliver a countershock to motion artifact. This leads to a restatement of one of the most important safety principles for operation of any automatic defibrillator: **There must be no movement of the patient or the device while the defibrillator is in its automatic or analyze mode.**

1. *Patient movement during transport.* Never attempt to analyze the rhythm during transport. The general rule is: Bring rescue vehicles to a complete stop before switching to automatic or analyze mode. This rule, of course, does not apply to air transport: either rotor craft or fixed wing. The effect of motion from air transport on the rhythm detector of the automatic defibrillators has not been studied extensively. The available evidence, however, suggests that aircraft motion during stable flight will *not* interfere with rhythm analysis by automatic defibrillators. Automatic rhythm analysis, unless absolutely required, should not be relied on during air transport.
2. *Agonal respirations.* The slow, gasping agonal respirations that often occur when a patient first goes into cardiac arrest pose a problem for AEDs. Agonal respirations at a rate of about seven or more per minute may prevent some automated defibrillators from entering the analyze mode, and the message "Stop all motion" or "Motion detected" will appear on the message screen. Similarly, with another automated defibrillator, movement from agonal respirations can produce artifact signals that interfere with rhythm analysis and may be misinterpreted. The rescuer must continue with CPR until the agonal respirations virtually cease; that is, they occur at a rate of four or less per minute.
3. *Continued chest compressions, ventilations, or other patient contact.* All contact between the patient and other personnel must cease while the rhythm is being analyzed. This includes such contacts as gently holding an oxygen mask against the patient's face or checking for the pulse.

Excessive 60-Hertz Interference

It is possible that 60-hertz interference from nearby electrical appliances may interfere with rhythm analysis by the automatic defibrillators. Electric blankets, fluorescent lights, and nearby clocks, radios, and television are the worst offenders. Electric blankets, in particular, if in contact with the patient, should be unplugged, or the patient should be moved to a different location.

Equipment Problems

There are a number of warning signals on the defibrillators to indicate low batteries, end of tape cassettes, loose electrodes, and so on. Several components of the defibrillators will occasionally produce such problems as blown fuses, paper recorders that jam and do not run, defective ECG paper styluses, and prolonged charge times. EMT-Ds should become thoroughly familiar with the operating manual of their defibrillator, so they can quickly recognize these problems and respond correctly.

Equipment Inspections

The mechanical integrity of a defibrillator should be checked regularly, following a standard checklist. This is the best guarantee that equipment problems will not occur in the field with patients in cardiac arrest. Manufacturers' recommendations will help determine the items in the equipment inspection checklist. Table 6–1 presents a sample checklist.

C. TROUBLESHOOTING PERSONNEL PERFORMANCE PROBLEMS

Two common performance problems are *slowness* and *failure to follow standard operating procedures.*

TABLE 6–1 Sample Checklist for Equipment Inspections

1. Inspect for general mechanical integrity.
2. Check patient monitor leads and cables.
3. Check quality of monitor display if present on AED.
4. Check all visual and audio indicator signals.
5. Run the tape recorder, provide a sample statement, and check that voice and rhythm are recorded. May use a rhythm simulator or a person.
6. Make sure that the batteries are adequately charged.
7. Check the presence and condition of accessories and supplies:
   a. Tape cassette
   b. Defibrillatory pads
   c. Disposable monitor leads, if needed to monitor with the specific AED
   d. Electrode gel, paste, or disposable pads, if needed
   e. Safety razor blade
   f. Towel and alcohol swabs

Slowness

The importance of rapid delivery of defibrillatory shocks has been emphasized repeatedly throughout this book. *Slowness,* regardless of its cause, must be considered a major performance problem. Slowness may have several causes:

1. *Lack of familiarity with equipment.* Rescuers must have frequent practice drills with their defibrillator so that all the steps involved in patient care occur smoothly and efficiently. Delays can occur while opening the packages for defibrillator pads, connecting the cables, placing the defibrillator pads, or responding to error messages.
2. *Mistaken priorities.* The rescuer who carries the defibrillator must attach and operate the device without delay. For a patient in cardiac arrest there is no activity, other than ensuring safety and obtaining sufficient room to work, that must be done before defibrillation. This includes basic CPR, endotracheal intubation, setting up oxygen supplies or suctioning equipment, attempts to analyze nonventricular fibrillation rhythms, long verbal reports, or taking the history from bystanders. If sufficient personnel are available, these activities should proceed simultaneously. However, with limited response teams, the highest priority should be given to defibrillation as early as possible.
3. *Lack of a sense of urgency.* Rescuers must tread a narrow path between a sense of urgency that leads to quick and efficient performance, and clumsy haste that leads to errors and mistakes. This is best achieved by regular practice drills that emphasize both correct performance and speed. EMT-Ds must not proceed casually through their standing orders. They should have a growing sense of discomfort with every second that passes without an electric countershock.

Failure to Follow Standard Operating Procedures

There are a number of operator errors in the use of automatic defibrillators that prevent delivery of a countershock to patients who have ventricular fibrillation. These must be considered serious, major errors and should prompt refresher training when they occur. The most common are:

1. Failure to place the devices in their automatic or analyze mode
2. Failure to allow sufficient time in automatic or analyze mode

3. Failure to press the shock button when the "shock-advised" message appears on the liquid-crystal display screen
4. Failure to avoid movement from CPR, agonal respirations, or contact with the patient
5. Failure to maintain equipment properly

In addition, there are other errors that are less serious in that they would not prevent delivery of a countershock to patients in ventricular fibrillation. These include:

1. Lack of an audible or adequate verbal report
2. Failure to record the event due to tape recorder problems such as recording on the tape leader, or unseated or misplaced tapes
3. Failure to provide a paper ECG recording of the rhythm
4. Taking long periods of time to proceed from step to step

APPENDICES

APPENDIX I	Essential Requirements for an Early Defibrillation Program
APPENDIX II	Standing Orders for Personnel Certified in Automated Defibrillation
APPENDIX III	For the Medical Director: Principles for Standing Orders for Automated Defibrillation Programs
APPENDIX IV	Bibliography of Articles and Books on Early Defibrillation
APPENDIX V	Training Curriculum for Automated Defibrillation

APPENDIX I

ESSENTIAL REQUIREMENTS FOR AN EARLY DEFIBRILLATION PROGRAM

1. *Basic certification as an EMT.* Satisfactory skills in basic life support, airway management, and patient assessment are prerequisites to enrollment in an EMT-D/first responder program.
2. *Medical director.* A medical doctor must assume responsibility for all prehospital medical care that involves EMT defibrillation.
3. *Patient-care protocols.* Standing orders must be approved and authorized by the local program medical director.
4. *State-EMS approved training program.* This program must include written and practical testing.
5. *Continuing-education program.* The minimum continuing-education requirement is a documented practical skills review performed at least every 90 days (3 months). Recertification must occur every 3 years.
6. *Dual-channel defibrillators.* Programs can only adopt manual, automatic, or semiautomatic defibrillators that are capable of recording both voice and the cardiac rhythm during a cardiac arrest.
7. *Written reports.* A written incident report must be provided on all prehospital care involving defibrillators. All programs must have ongoing data collection that includes case-by-case review of performance and analyses over time of program outcomes.
8. *Satisfactory performance.* The EMT-D/first responder must perform within the guidelines provided by the program's medical director and confirmed by medical review of every patient by either the program medical director or his or her designated representative.

APPENDIX II

STANDING ORDERS FOR PERSONNEL CERTIFIED IN AUTOMATED DEFIBRILLATION

TO:	King County defibrillation-certified emergency personnel
FROM:	Richard O. Cummins, M.D., Medical Director, King County EMT Defibrillation Program
DATE:	August 1, 1988
SCOPE:	These standing orders go into effect August 1, 1988, and replace all previous standing orders for defibrillation-certified EMTs/first responders.
PURPOSE	The purpose of these orders is to provide prompt defibrillation for patients who have confirmed circulatory arrest due to ventricular fibrillation.
AUTHORIZATION:	In the event of a cardiac arrest in King County, you are authorized to perform the following:

1. Immediately upon arrival, verify circulatory and respiratory arrest by the absence of normal consciousness, normal respirations, and carotid pulse.
2. Initiate CPR and the defibrillation protocol.
3. DEFIBRILLATION PROTOCOL: Certified emergency personnel in King County are authorized to deliver up to six electric countershocks with an automated defibrillator to ventricular fibrillation. This should be done as quickly as possible, with a minimum interruption of CPR. Exact details of sequencing can vary as long as the following overall goals are realized:
    a. Ventricular fibrillation (and only VF) is shocked repeatedly and as fast as possible.
    b. CPR is interrupted for a minimum of time.
    c. Overall patient care and safety are never neglected.
4. ASSESSMENT: Assess the rhythm for the presence of ventricular fibrillation:
    a. Turn defibrillator power ON (and recorder ON if controlled separately).
    b. Begin verbal report.
    c. Attach defibrillator pads.
    d. Clear the patient (stop CPR).
    e. Switch to AUTO or to ANALYZE mode.
    f. Count to 15 seconds.

5. TREATMENT: Treat ventricular fibrillation with a maximum of six countershocks.
    a. When ventricular fibrillation is persistent, you may deliver up to three shocks without stopping between shocks to administer CPR.
    b. Press the SHOCK control when so indicated, or allow the AUTO mode to deliver the shock.
    c. Allow the device to continue to assess and treat for up to three shocks in a row.
    d. Whenever a 15-second assessment period occurs without a shock, switch to MANUAL mode and resume CPR for 15 to 30 seconds.
    e. Switch back to AUTO mode and allow the device to assess and treat for up to three more shocks in a row.

Details of Standing Orders for Patient Treatment

1. *Two-person response team.* One EMT/first responder initiates one-person CPR using pocket face mask ventilations, and continues this role throughout the resuscitation. The other EMT becomes the "defibrillator EMT," directing the resuscitation and operating the defibrillator. The defibrillator EMT is in charge of the scene and of patient care.
2. *Three-person-or-more response teams.* Two EMTs/first responders initiate two-person CPR using the bag-valve mask or the pocket face mask, and continue this role throughout the resuscitation. The other EMT becomes the "defibrillator EMT," directing the resuscitation and operating the defibrillator. The defibrillator EMT is in charge of the scene and of patient care.
3. *No prescribed period of initial CPR.* Upon arrival at the scene and verification of cardiac arrest, the defibrillator EMT does not wait for CPR to be performed for any set period of time, but proceeds immediately with the defibrillation protocols outlined in these standing orders.
4. *No excessive interruptions of CPR.* If delays in CPR of 5 seconds or more are encountered due to battery problems, artifact troubleshooting, uncertainty of rhythm, and so on, resume CPR until the problem is resolved. Then reassess. Delays in CPR for more than 5 seconds are permitted only during the assessment period by the automatic defibrillator. In particular: Do not delay CPR while checking to see if a rhythm is producing a pulse. **Pulse checks should take no more than 5 seconds. If no pulse in 5 seconds, resume CPR immediately.**

5. *Blood pressure less than 60.* If the patient's systolic blood pressure is less than 60 mmHg, and the patient remains unconscious, continue CPR. Do not stop chest compressions just because the heart has started to beat. The beat may be inadequate for survival but still give a palpable pulse. Do not depend on palpation to measure the blood pressure—it is notoriously inaccurate.
6. *Maximum of 15-second assessment periods.* Automated defibrillators should be left in AUTO mode or ANALYZE mode no longer than 15 seconds except for two situations:
   a. The device is delivering stacked shocks.
   b. The device begins to charge. If the charging alarm is heard, allow that treatment cycle to be completed.
7. *Rapid defibrillation.* The first shock should be delivered within 60 to 90 seconds of the emergency personnel's arrival at the patient's side. Defibrillation is of extremely high priority in a cardiac arrest. It takes precedence over history taking and the verbal report, and should proceed simultaneously with basic CPR, airway maintenance, and oxygenation. Never delay rhythm assessment and defibrillation to troubleshoot problems with the tape cassette or to provide hyperventilation or a prescribed period of CPR.
8. *Verbal report.* The recorder must be turned on throughout the resuscitation attempt.
   a. Identify yourself and the responding fire department.
   b. Briefly describe the situation.
   c. Report each step as you proceed through the standing orders.
   d. Continue to report events as they occur.
9. *Defibrillator pad attachment for automated defibrillators.* Upon verification of cardiac arrest, defibrillator pads (only) should be attached. Verbally identify their positions: "one to the right sternal border, and one to the apex regions of the heart."
10. *Age and weight guidelines.* Children under the age of 12 should not be defibrillated by emergency personnel *unless* they weigh at least 90 pounds. If a person is in ventricular fibrillation and age and weight are in these approximate ranges, countershocks should be delivered per the regular standing orders.

APPENDIX III

FOR THE MEDICAL DIRECTOR: PRINCIPLES FOR STANDING ORDERS FOR AUTOMATED DEFIBRILLATION PROGRAMS

Each program's medical director may decide on slight variations in the local standing orders. Treatment protocols may vary in terms of CPR administration, total number of allowed shocks, the energy levels of the countershocks, and the treatment approach to other rhythms. Several principles guide the development of the standing orders. If these principles are understood, each program's medical director can develop a suitable local protocol:

1. An automated defibrillator must be properly attached *to the patient* and then be given time (usually 15 seconds) to assess the rhythm, charge the capacitors if ventricular fibrillation is present, and deliver a shock. During this period, *all* contact with the patient must cease.
2. The whole idea of the standing orders is to "sandwich" the AED assessments periods between periods of ongoing CPR.
3. Therefore, the medical director must decide:
    a. How much CPR and patient care should occur both *before* and *between* the AED assessments.
    b. How many total assessments the AED is going to have.
4. What makes the standing orders relatively complicated is the fact that the AED can do one of two things during each AED assessment period—it will either charge and deliver a countershock, or it will do nothing. In addition, *three* things can happen following each countershock:
    a. The rhythm will remain in ventricular fibrillation.
    b. The rhythm will change to a perfusing rhythm.
    c. The rhythm will change to a nonperfusing rhythm that is not ventricular fibrillation.
5. Successful use of an automatic defibrillator still requires two major assessments by the EMT(s):
    a. Was a shock actually delivered?
    b. Does the patient now have a perfusing rhythm that results in an adequate blood pressure?

Most experienced early defibrillation programs have made the following decisions about the use of an automated defibrillator:

1. Defibrillatory pads should be placed only on people in *full* cardiac arrest.
2. There should be no *required* period of CPR before attachment and use of the AED. Deployment of an AED requires about 45 to 60 seconds. Therefore, all patients will receive approximately 1 minute of CPR prior to any countershocks.
3. For persistent ventricular fibrillation, a total of six defibrillatory shocks can be given. If the rhythm remains ventricular fibrillation after three shocks, King County EMTs stop assessments with the AED and perform CPR for 15 to 30 seconds. They then deliver three more shocks. If ventricular fibrillation remains after six shocks, they continue CPR until the arrival of the paramedics. In systems without a tiered response the EMTs must transport the patients to a distant emergency facility. In these settings the medical director may decide to permit additional countershocks to refractory ventricular fibrillation.
4. Pulse checks always come after a period of CPR, not immediately after an assessment/treatment period by the AED. This approach minimizes the time without CPR and is easier for the responders to remember.

APPENDIX IV

BIBLIOGRAPHY OF ARTICLES AND BOOKS ON EARLY DEFIBRILLATION*

ADVANCED CORONARY TREATMENT FOUNDATION. "Medical Advisory Board Statement on EMT-Defibrillation," *Journal of Emergency Medical Services,* November 1983, 8:37.

AMERICAN COLLEGE OF EMERGENCY PHYSICIANS EMS COMMITTEE. "Prehospital Defibrillation by Basic-Level Emergency Medical Technicians," *Annals of Emergency Medicine,* October 1984, 13:10.

AMERICAN HEART ASSOCIATION. "Standards and Guidelines for Cardiopulmonary Resuscitation and Emergency Cardiac Care," *Journal of the American Medical Association,* June 1986.

ANDRESEN, E. "Home Defibrillators for High Risk Cardiac Patients," *Caring,* February 1987, 6(2):32–35.

APPLEBAUM, D. "The Introduction of Automatic External Defibrillation to a Basic Ambulance System in Israel," *PACE,* 1988, 11:884(abs).

ARONSON, A. L. AND HAGGAR, B. "The Automatic Defibrillator-Pacemaker: Clinical Rational and Engineering Design," *Medical Instrumentation,* 1986, 20:27–35.

ATKINS, J. M. "Emergency Medical Service Systems in Acute Cardiac Care: State of the Art," *Circulation,* 1986, 74 (suppl IV):4.

ATKINS, J. M., MURPHY, D. M., ALLISON, E. J. AND GRAVES, J. R. "Toward Earlier Defibrillation," *Journal of Emergency Medical Services,* June 1986, 11:70.

BACHMAN, J. W., MCDONALD, G. S. AND O'BRIEN, P. "A Study of Out-of-Hospital Cardiac Arrests in Northeastern Minnesota," *Journal of the American Medical Association,* 1986, 256(4):477–83.

BRADLEY, K., SOKOLOW, A. E., WRIGHT, K. J. AND MCCULLOUGH, W. J. "A Comparison of an Innovative Four-Hour EMT-D Course with a 'Standard' 10-Hour Course," *Annals of Emergency Medicine,* 1988, 17:613–19.

BERGNER, L., HALLSTROM, A. P., BERGNER, M., EISENBERG, M. S. AND COBB, L. A. "Service Factors and Health Status of Survivors of Out-of-Hospital Cardiac Arrest," *American Journal of Emergency Medicine,* 1983, 1:259–63.

BUNTING-BLAKE, L., PARKER, J., WEIGEL, A. AND WHITE, R.D. *Defibrillation: A Manual for the EMT.* Philadelphia: J. B. Lippincott, 1985.

CHADDA, K. D., BARRY, M. F. AND KAMMERER, R. J. "Patient and Family Initiated Treatment for Out-of-Hospital Ventricular Tachyarrhythmias," *Circulation,* 1987, 76(suppl IV):12.

CHADDA, K. D. AND KAMMERER R. "Early Experiences with the Portable Automatic External Defibrillator in the Home and Public Places," *American Journal of Cardiology,* 1987, 60:732–33.

*Modified from a bibliography of articles on early defibrillation prepared by Mary Newman for the Citizen CPR Foundation, Inc.

CHADDA, K. D. AND KAMMERER, R. "Patient and Family Acceptance of Home Defibrillation and CPR Programs," *Circulation,* 1984, 70(suppl II):463.

CHADDA, K., KAMMERER, R., KUPHAL, J. AND MILLER, K. "Successful Defibrillation in the Industrial, Recreational and Corporate Settings by Laypersons," *Circulation,* 1987, 76(suppl IV):12.

CLYDE, C., KERR, A., VARGHESE, A. AND WILSON, C. "Defibrillators in General Practice," *British Medical Journal,* 17 November 1984, 289(6455):1351–53.

COPASS, M., EISENBERG, M. S. AND DAMON, S. *EMT-Defibrillation.* Westport, CT: ETI Publishers, 1984.

CUMMINS, R. O. "EMT Defibrillation: National Guidelines for Implementation," *American Journal of Emergency Medicine,* May 1987, 5(3):254–57.

CUMMINS, R. O. AND AUSTIN, D. A., JR. "The Frequency of 'Occult' Ventricular Fibrillation Masquerading as a Flat Line in Prehospital Cardiac Arrest," *Annals of Emergency Medicine,* 1988, 17:813–17.

CUMMINS, R. O., AUSTIN, D. A., JR., GRAVES, J. R. AND HAMBLEY, C. "An Innovative Approach to Medical Control: Semi-automatic Defibrillators with Solid State Memory Modules for Recording Cardiac Events," *Annals of Emergency Medicine,* 1988, 17:818–24.

CUMMINS, R. O. AND EISENBERG, M. S. "EMT Defibrillation: A Proven Concept," *American Heart Association Emergency Cardiac Care National Faculty Newsletter,* October 1984, 1:1–3.

CUMMINS, R. O., EISENBERG, M. S., BERGNER, L., HALLSTROM, A. P., HEARNE, T. AND MURRAY, J. A. "Automatic External Defibrillation: Evaluation of Its Role in the Home and in Emergency Medical Services," *Annals of Emergency Medicine,* September 1984, 13(9, Pt 2):789–801.

CUMMINS, R. O., EISENBERG, M. S., GRAVES, J. R., ET AL. "EMT-Defibrillation: Is It Right for You?" *Journal of Emergency Medical Services,* January 1985, 10:48–53.

CUMMINS, R. O., EISENBERG, M. S., GRAVES, J. R., AUSTIN, D. AND DAMON, S. "EMT-Defibrillation: Achieving Medical Control," *Journal of Emergency Medical Services,* March 1985, 10:45–53.

CUMMINS, R. O., EISENBERG, M. S., GRAVES, J. R., HEARNE, T., LITWIN, P. E. AND HALLSTROM, A. P. "Automatic External Defibrillators Used by Emergency Medical Technicians: A Controlled Clinical Trial," *Circulation,* 1985, 72(4): 111–18.

CUMMINS, R. O., EISENBERG, M. S., HALLSTROM, A. P., HEARNE, T. R., GRAVES, J. R. AND LITWIN, P. E. "What is a Save? Outcome Measures in Clinical Evaluations of Automatic External Defibrillators," *American Heart Journal,* December 1985, 110(6):1133–38.

CUMMINS, R. O., EISENBERG, M. S., LITWIN, P. E., GRAVES, J. R., HEARNE, T. R. AND HALLSTROM, A. P. "Automatic External Defibrillators Used by Emergency Medical Technicians," *Journal of the American Medical Association,* March 27, 1987, 257(12):1605–10.

CUMMINS, R. O., EISENBERG, M. S., MOORE, J. D., HEARNE, T. R., ANDRESEN, E., WENDT, R., LITWIN, P. E., GRAVES, J. R., HALLSTROM, A. P. AND PIERCE, J. "Automatic External Defibrillators: Clinical, Training, Psychological and Public Health Issues," *Annals of Emergency Medicine,* August 1985, 14(8):755–60.

CUMMINS, R. O., EISENBERG, M. S. AND STULTS, K. R. "Automatic External Defibrillators: Clinical Issues for Cardiology," *Circulation,* 1986, 73:381.

CUMMINS, R. O., GRAVES, J. R., EISENBERG, M. S., DAMON, S. AND PIERCE, J. "Implementing EMT-Defibrillation," *Journal of Emergency Medical Services,* February 1985, 10:44–47.

CUMMINS, R. O., STULTS, K. R., HAGGAR, B., KERBER, R. E., SCHAEFFER, S. AND BROWN, D. D. "A New Rhythm Library for Testing Automatic External Defibrillators: Performance of Three Devices," *Journal of the American College of Cardiology,* 1988, 11:597–602.

DALZELL, G. W. N., CUNNINGHAM, S. R., ALLEN, J. D., ANDERSON, J. AND ADGEY, A. J. "Ventricular Defibrillation: The Belfast Experience," *British Heart Journal,* November 1986, 58(5):441–46.

DIACK, A. W., WELBORN, W. S., RULLMAN, R. G. AND WAYNE, M. "An Automatic Cardiac Resuscitator for Emergency Treatment of Cardiac Arrest," *Medical Instrumentation,* 1979, 13:78.

EISENBERG, M. S. "Cardiopulmonary Resuscitation and Defibrillation," *Western Journal of Medicine,* 1987, 146(5):608–9.

EISENBERG, M. S., BERGNER, L. AND HALLSTROM, A. P. "Paramedic Programs and Out-of-Hospital Cardiac Arrest. I. Factors Associated with Successful Resuscitation," *American Journal of Public Health,* 1979, 69:3–38.

EISENBERG, M. S., BERGNER, L. AND HALLSTROM, A. P. "Paramedic Programs and Out-of-Hospital Cardiac Arrest. II. Impact on Community Mortality," *American Journal of Public Health,* 1979, 69:39–42.

EISENBERG, M. S., COPASS, M. K. AND HALLSTROM, A. P., ET AL. "Management of Out-of-Hospital Cardiac Arrest: Failure of Basic Emergency Medical Technician Services," *Journal of the American Medical Association,* 1980, 243: 1049–51.

EISENBERG, M. S., COPASS, M. K., HALLSTROM, A. P., BLAKE, B., BERGNER, L., SHORT, F. AND COBB, L. "Treatment of Out-of-Hospital Cardiac Arrest with Rapid Defibrillation by Emergency Medical Technicians," *New England Journal of Medicine,* 1980, 302:1379–83.

EISENBERG, M. S. AND CUMMINS, R. O. "Automatic External Defibrillation: Bringing It Home," editorial, *American Journal of Emergency Medicine,* November 1985, 3(6):568–69.

EISENBERG, M. S. AND CUMMINS, R. O. "Defibrillation Performed by the Emergency Medical Technician," *Circulation,* December 1986, 74(6 Pt 2) (suppl IV):9–12.

EISENBERG, M. S. AND CUMMINS, R. O. "EMT Defibrillation," letter, *Annals of Emergency Medicine,* May 1985, 14(5):487.

EISENBERG, M. S., CUMMINS, R. O., HALLSTROM, A. P. AND HEARNE, T. "Defibrillation by Emergency Medical Technicians," *Critical Care Medicine,* 1985, 13(11):921–22.

EISENBERG, M. S., HALLSTROM, A. P., COPASS, M. K., BERGNER, L., SHORT, F. AND PIERCE, J. "Treatment of Ventricular Fibrillation: Emergency Medical Technician Defibrillation and Paramedic Services," *Journal of the American Medical Association,* 1984, 251(13):1723–26.

ESTELL, D. A. AND SMOCK, S. N. "Blind Defibrillation outside the Hospital," *Journal of the American College of Emergency Physicians,* July 1976, 5(7):512–14.

FORSTER, F. K. AND WEAVER, W. D. "Automatic Recognition of Ventricular Fibrillation and Other Rhythms in Patients Developing Cardiac Arrest," *IEEE Computer Society, Computers in Cardiology,* 1983; 245–48.

GRAVES, J. R. AND CUMMINS, R. O. "Defibrillation by EMT's," in Heckman, J. D., editor. *Emergency Care and Transportation of the Sick and Injured,* 4th Ed., Appendix C. Chicago: American Academy of Orthopedic Surgeons, 1987.

GRAY, A. J., REDMOND, A. D. AND MARTIN, M. A. "Use of the Automatic External Defibrillator-Pacemaker by Ambulance Personnel: The Stockport Experience," *British Medical Journal,* May 2, 1987, 294(6580):1133–35.

HALLSTROM, A. P., EISENBERG, M. S. AND BERGNER, L. "The Potential Use of Automatic Defibrillators in the Home for Management of Cardiac Arrest," *Medical Care,* 1984, 22(12):1083–87.

HAUSWALD, M. "Defibrillation in the Field: Should EMT's Interpret Rhythms?" *American Journal of Emergency Medicine,* May 1986, 4(3):274–75.

JACK, C. M., HUNTER, E. K., PRINGLE, T. H., WILSON, J. T., ANDERSON, J. AND ADGEY, A. J. "An External Automatic Device to Detect Ventricular Fibrillation," *European Heart Journal,* 1986, 7:404–11.

JACK, C. M., HUNTER, E. K., PRINGLE, T. H., WILSON, J. T., ANDERSON, J. AND ADGEY, A. J. "Automatic Detection of Cardiac Arrest Rhythms Prior to Automatic External Cardiac Defibrillation," *Texas Heart Institute Journal,* 1986, 13:419–26.

JACOS, L. "Medical, Legal and Social Implications of Automatic External Defibrillators," *Annals of Emergency Medicine,* 1986, 15:863–64.

JAGGARAO, N. S., GRAINGER, R., HEBER, M., VINCENT, R. AND CHAMBERLAIN, R. "Use of an Automated External Defibrillator-Pacemaker by Ambulance Staff," *Lancet,* 1982, ii:73–75.

JAKOBSSON, J., NYQUIST, O. AND REHNQUIST, N. "Effects of Early Defibrillation of Out-of-Hospital Cardiac Arrest Patients by Ambulance Personnel," *European Heart Journal,* November 1987, 8(11):1189–94.

JAKOBSSON, J., NYQUIST, O., REHNQUIST, N. AND NORBERG, K. "Cost of a Saved Life Following Out-of-Hospital Cardiac Arrest Resuscitated by Specially Trained Ambulance Personnel," *Acta Anaesthesiologica Scandinavica,* 1987, 31:426–29.

MOORE, J. E., EISENBERG, M. S., CUMMINS, R. O., HALLSTROM, A., LITWIN, P. AND CARTER, W. "Lay Person Use of Automatic External Defibrillation," *Annals of Emergency Medicine,* June 1987, 16(6):669–72.

MURPHY, D. M. "EMT-D: Finding the Right Combination," *Journal of Emergency Medical Services,* May 1984, 9:46–49.

MURPHY, D. M. "Rapid Defibrillation: Fire Service to Lead the Way," *Journal of Emergency Medical Services,* June 1987, 12:67–71.

NEWMAN, M. M. "Advancing Resuscitation Abroad," *Journal of Emergency Medical Services,* November 1987, 12:22–26.

NEWMAN, M. M. "EMT-D Standards," *Journal of Emergency Medical Services,* June 1986, 11:68–70.

NEWMAN, M. M. "National EMT-D Study," *Journal of Emergency Medical Services,* July 1986, 11:70–72.

NEWMAN, M. M. "The Survival Advantage: Early Defibrillation Programs in the Fire Service," *Journal of Emergency Medical Services,* June 1987, 12:40–46.

OLSON, D. W., LAROCHELLE, J., FARK, D., MILBRATH, M., HENDLET, G., AUFDERHEIDE, T., ET AL. "EMT-D: The Wisconsin Experience," *Annals of Emergency Medicine,* 1988, 16:944. (abs).

ORNATO, J. P., CRAREN, E. J., GONZALEZ, E. R., GARNETT, A. R., MCKLUNG, B. K. AND NEWMAN, M. M. "Cost Effectiveness of Defibrillation by Emergency Medical Technicians," *American Journal of Emergency Medicine,* March 1988, 6(2):108–12.

ORNATO, J. P., MCNEIL, S. E., CRAREN, E. J., ET AL. "Limitations on Effectiveness of Rapid Defibrillation by Emergency Medical Technicians in a Rural Setting," *Annals of Emergency Medicine,* 1984, 13:1096–99.

PARIS, P. M. "EMT-Defibrillation: A Recipe for Saving Lives," *American Journal of Emergency Medicine,* 1988, 6:282–87.

PIERCE, J., WENDT, R. W., ANDRESEN, E., HEARNE, T. R., EISENBERG, M. S., CUMMINS, R. O., LITWIN, P. E. AND HALLSTROM, A. P. "Automatic External Defibrillation: Lay Person Use in the Home," *Journal of Emergency Medical Services,* March 1986, 11(3):58–60.

ROSE, L. B. AND PRESS, E. "Cardiac Defibrillation by Ambulance Attendants," *Journal of the American Medical Association,* 1972, 219(1):63–68.

ROZKOVEC, A., CROSSLEY, J., WALESBY, R., FOX, K. M. AND MASERI, A. "Safety and Effectiveness of a Portable External Automatic Defibrillator-Pacemaker," *Clinical Cardiology,* 1983, 6:527–33.

STULTS, K. R. "Automatic and Semi-automatic Defibrillation," Appendix in Grant, H. D., Murray, R. H., Bergeron, J. D., *Emergency Care,* 4th Ed., Revised. Englewood Cliffs, NJ: Prentice Hall (a Brady book), 1988.

STULTS, K. R. "EMT Defibrillation in Rural America," *Physician Assistant,* September 1986, 10(9):11–12, 117, 120–21.

STULTS, K. R. *EMT-D Prehospital Defibrillation.* Englewood Cliffs, NJ: Prentice Hall (a Brady book), 1986.

STULTS, K. R. "Phone First," *Journal of Emergency Medical Services,* September 1987, 12:28.

STULTS, K. R. "Statewide Efforts to Improve Survival from Out-of-Hospital Cardiac Arrest," *Journal of Iowa Medical Society,* April 1985, 75(4).

STULTS, K. R. AND BROWN, D. D. "Refibrillation Managed by EMT-D's: Incidence and Outcome without Paramedic Backup," *American Journal of Emergency Medicine,* 1986, 4(6):491–95.

STULTS, K. R. AND BROWN, D. D. "Special Considerations for Defibrillation Performed by Emergency Medical Technicians in Small Communities," *Circulation,* 1986, 74(suppl IV):13–17.

STULTS, K. R., BROWN, D. D., COOLEY, F. AND KERBER, R. E. "Self-Adhesive Monitor-Defibrillator Pads Improve Prehospital Defibrillation Success," *Annals of Emergency Medicine,* August 1987, 16:872–77.

STULTS, K. R., BROWN, D. D. AND KERBER, R. E. "Efficacy of an Automated External Defibrillator in the Management of Out-of-Hospital Cardiac Arrest: Validation of the Diagnostic Algorithm and Initial Clinical Experience in a Rural Environment," *Circulation,* 1986, 73(4):701–9.

STULTS, K. R., BROWN, D. D. AND KERBER, R. E. "Self-Adhesive Monitor-Defibrillator Pads: Prehospital Use," *Journal of the American College of Cardiology,* 1986, 7(2):241.

STULTS, K. R., BROWN, D. D., SCHUG, V. L. AND BEAN, J. A. "Prehospital Defibrillation by Emergency Medical Technicians: Reply," *New England Journal of Medicine,* 310(23):1533.

STULTS, K. R., BROWN, D. D., SCHUG, V. L. AND BEAN, J. A. "Prehospital Defibrillation Performed by Emergency Medical Technicians in Rural Communities," *New England Journal of Medicine,* 1984, 310:219–23.

STULTS, K. R. AND CUMMINS, R. O. "Fully Automatic vs. Shock Advisory Defibrillators: What Are the Issues?" *Journal of Emergency Medical Services,* September 1987, 12:71–73.

STULTS, K. R., CUMMINS, R. O., WHITE, R. D. AND GRAVES, J. R. "Making EMT-D Work: Proceedings from the University of Iowa Workshop, Parts I and II," *Journal of Emergency Medical Services,* February 1986, 11(2):26–32 and March 1986, 11(3):50–56.

SWENSON, R. D., HILL, D. L., MARTIN, J. S., WIRKUS, M. AND WEAVER, W. D. "Automatic External Defibrillators Used by Family Members to Treat Cardiac Arrest," *Circulation,* 1987, 76(suppl IV):463.

VUKOV, L. F., WHITE, R. D. AND BACKMAN, J. W. "New Perspectives on Rural EMT Defibrillation," *Annals of Emergency Medicine,* April 1988, 17(4):318–21.

WEAVER, W. D., COPASS, M. K. AND COBB, L. A. "Early Defibrillation in a City Having Paramedic Services: A Preliminary Report," *European Heart Journal,* 1983, 4:98.

WEAVER, W. D., COPASS, M. K. AND COBB, L. A. "Early Defibrillation of Cardiac Arrest Victims by Trained Basic Life Support Providers in a City Having Paramedic Services," *Clinical Research,* 1982, 30(1):23.

WEAVER, W. D., COPASS, M. K. AND COBB, L. A. "Improved Neurologic Recovery and Survival after Early Defibrillation," *Circulation,* 1984, 69(5):943–48.

WEAVER, W.D., COPASS, M. K., HILL, D. L., FAHRENBRUCH, C., HALLSTROM, A. P. AND COBB, L. A. "Cardiac Arrest Treated with a New Automatic External

Defibrillator by Out-of-Hospital First Responders," *American Journal of Cardiology,* 1986, 57:1017–21.

WEAVER, W.D., HILL, D. L., COPASS, M. K., ET AL. "Improved Survival Rates from Cardiac Arrest Using Automatic External Defibrillators," *Circulation,* 1985, 72(suppl III):8.

WEAVER, W.D., RAY, R., COBB, L. A., BUFI, D. AND HALLSTROM, A. P. "Early Defibrillation for Out-of-Hospital Cardiac Arrest," *Circulation,* 1983, 68(4):14.

WEIGEL, A. "EMT-D or EMT-P: Who's Got the Joules?" *Journal of Emergency Medical Services,* July 1986, 11:5–6.

WEIGEL, A., ATKINS, J. M. AND TAYLOR, J. *Automated Defibrillation.* Englewood, CO: Morton Publishing Company, 1988.

WHITE, R. D. "EMT-Defibrillation: Time for Controlled Implementation of Effective Treatment," *American Heart Association Emergency Cardiac Care National Faculty Newsletter,* 1986, 8:1–3.

APPENDIX V

TRAINING CURRICULUM FOR AUTOMATED DEFIBRILLATION*

Introduction

This curriculum outlines the automated defibrillation class used in King County, Washington. It is written to the course instructor but is meant to be useful to those program medical directors and EMS administrators wondering just how to go about putting together a course based on national EMT-D standards. It answers these concerns:

1. How to use the 4 to 6 hours recommended for class time
2. How to set up practical sessions for best learning psychomotor skills
3. What parts of the class are best taught by the physician medical director
4. What audiovisuals are most useful
5. What role the instructors should play and what their qualifications should be
6. What books are most helpful for "automatic defibrillation" training
7. What kinds of instructional equipment needs to be assembled and in what quantity
8. How to test for skill competency

We think this curriculum, which we learned by trial and error while teaching more than 600 rescuers to operate automatic defibrillators, will help others to start early defibrillation programs smoothly.

Instructional Principles

Despite the apparent simplicity of automatic and semiautomatic defibrillators, a well-organized training program must include operation, application, maintenance, and troubleshooting the device. The major difference between a rescuer who is trained to defibrillate using a standard manual device and one trained to use an automated defibrillator is the ability to interpret ECG rhythms. The course is designed

*This curriculum for initial training for early defibrillation programs is consistent with the National Standards for EMT Defibrillation developed by the National Council for State Emergency Medical Services Training Coordinators.

around this principle: early defibrillation is a psychomotor skill, to be performed quickly and smoothly much in the same manner as CPR skills. Often, the rescuer must perform this skill under adverse conditions without hesitation—almost as a reflexive action. Training is aimed toward competent performance that measures student success. Performance failures have been rare and without exception were corrected by individual instruction and additional practice.

Instructional Approach

1. Varied instructional techniques worked best since students learned the skill in different ways. Included are demonstrations, lectures, slide presentations, reading materials, practice time with and without supervision, and simulated cardiac arrest scenarios.
2. The practical skills of defibrillation are the core of each class segment. Students see and perform the skill many times throughout the class. This develops familiarity with equipment and standing orders.
3. Both classes use small-group teaching stations equipped for practicing defibrillation. There is a ratio of one instructor for every six students. Instructors can be experienced EMT-Ds or paramedics. (see instructor qualifications) Most learning seems to "solidify" during practical sessions.
4. The concept of electrocardiology is introduced, but rhythm recognition is not required. Most rescuers learn basic dying heart rhythms through exposure and individual interest.
5. Machine maintenance composes one segment in the practical teaching stations.
6. Standing orders provide the nucleus for this curriculum. The student must know standing orders by heart.
7. This course assumes that emergency personnel have had a review of BCLS. If the medical director is concerned about basic skills, we suggest an optional screening evaluation conducted prior to the course to locate students who have become "rusty" on their CPR and airway maintenance skills.

Course Objectives

At the end of this course, the student will demonstrate competency with a written test scoring 80 percent or better and a practical test managing a cardiac arrest patient using defibrillation.

Written test. The written test includes the following five behavioral objectives:

1. The student will identify the function, operation, and proper maintenance of the AED/SAED.
2. The student will define patient assessment, and care and treatment of the sudden death victim.
3. The student will list safety measures when using an AED/SAED.
4. The student will repeat standing orders and local EMT-D program requirements.
5. The student will document a cardiac arrest call using local procedures.

Practical test. The practical test contains the following five behavioral objectives:

1. The student will demonstrate control of the emergency scene and will direct the resuscitation efforts.
2. The student will demonstrate correct use of standing orders in a simulated cardiac arrest by correctly defibrillating a manikin within 90 seconds of arrival at the manikin's side.
3. The student will demonstrate safe use of the AED/SAED and answer questions about the controls, disposable supplies, and maintenance, and will devise troubleshooting techniques.
4. The student will give an appropriate voice documentation of events on the scene.
5. The student will demonstrate appropriate assessment and care of the patient before, during, and after defibrillation.

Course Prerequisites

1. *Proof of current EMT or first-responder status.* If EMT certification expires, EMT-D certification also lapses until the EMT is recertified. (If the early defibrillation program is part of a fire service Rapid Zap program, the student must present proof that he or she is currently in good standing with that program's requirements.)
2. *Approval to enroll* from the student's program director (fire chief, medical control officer, or other person responsible for the rescuer's professional performance).

3. *Proof of current basic cardiac life-support skills* (an AHA or Red Cross card). These skills will be tested along with the rescuer's skills at the time of the written and practical exam. Any student not performing BCLS to AHA standards will have authorization to defibrillate withheld until he or she achieves competency in BCLS.
   a. In general, the student must come to the class with satisfactory knowledge of patient assessment and all basic life-support information and skills.
   b. In particular, this includes proper use of all ventilatory adjuncts that may be used, including oropharyngeal airways, bag valve mask, or pocket face mask.

Student Materials

A folder that contains the following material is prepared for each student:

1. Registration form
2. Standing orders from the local medical director
3. List of certification and recertification requirements
4. List of medical–legal requirements of state and local program
5. Check sheet for final practical exam
6. Supplemental student study guide to cardiac anatomy and electrophysiology
7. Operation and maintenance instructions for the selected service defibrillator (generally photocopied, with permission, from the operating manual of each defibrillator manufacturer)
8. (*Optional*) Textbook on EMT/first responder defibrillation
9. Course evaluation form

Class Equipment

Student packets enough for each student

Written exams for each student

Lesson plan (copies for all instructors)

Textbook for each student

Slide projector (if lecture includes slides) with carousel, screen, extension cord, remote control extension cord, and at least one extra bulb

Equipment needed for every six students:

- List of scenarios to be practiced in the small group
- One resuscitation manikin
- One defibrillator, with cables, disposable pads, and battery-charging unit
- One arrhythmia simulator, plus spare batteries
- One pocket face mask

Disposable supplies:

- Manikin cleaning supplies
- Disposable razors
- Extra disposable defibrillator pads
- Armoral (keeps adhesive pads from adhering to manikin chest plate)
- ECG paper (if needed for the defibrillator)
- Cassette recording tapes
- Monitoring equipment, if applicable

Course Overview: Suggested Use of Class Time

AED/SAED training requires a total of 4 to 6 hours. The most effective learning and skill retention appears to occur when the training is divided into two classes of 2 to 3 hours each. It is quite practical to divide the training into two sessions that occur on the same day. Our experience suggests that two classes at least one day apart are optimal, but not essential.

Class 1 (2 to 3 hours in length)

Time	Elapsed	
:15		Introduction and paperwork
:15	:30	Introductory comments from medical director
:15	:45	Demonstration 1: the standing orders
:15	1:00	Demonstration 2: the defibrillator
:15	1:15	Demonstration 3: cardiac arrest!
:45	2:00	Small-group practice: using a defibrillator
:15	2:15	Whole-class question-and-answer session

Class 2 (2 to 3 hours)

Time	Elapsed	
:30		Medical control and the EMT/first responder: lecture by the medical director or program coordinator
:15	:45	Troubleshooting the device: "a dead defibrillator means a dead patient"
1:00	1:45	Small-group practice: practical hands-on time in small groups with instructors
:30–?	2:15–?	Written and practical testing: all practice stations remain open until all students complete testing: students are allowed to review and retest up to three times

Course Overview: Suggested Content

Class 1. The first session includes introduction to the program, demonstrations of the skills to be learned, review of sudden cardiac death, introduction to specific defibrillator used by the service, and practice by each student of the skills of defibrillation. This class is designed to demystify automatic defibrillation. The student will have a clear view of what is expected in testing situations and in the field. The didactic portion is brief. The major concept imparted in electrocardiology is the difference in an *ECG rhythm* and an actual *pulse.* Most rescuers go on their own to learn peri-arrest rhythms. Emphasis is placed on maintenance of the defibrillator and learning all controls. Considerable time is allotted to students' hands on the machine. They should leave this class with an understanding of defibrillation and a working knowledge of the AED/SAED they will be using.

Class 2. The second session begins with another demonstration emphasizing standing orders. Didactic portion includes details of documentation, local program requirements, and treating the patient before, during, and after implementing defibrillation standing orders. In the troubleshooting portion of this class instructors demonstrate what could possibly happen at the scene of a cardiac arrest, including device problems and scene hazards. The bulk of this class is in small-group practicals, where the rescuers in small groups practice and evaluate one another's performance in varied simulated situations. Class ends with written and practical tests.

This class consolidates the student skills and prepares the student for the challenges they must face in the field. Prior to testing, the instructors should be fairly confident that students are prepared to be evaluated. Plenty of time is allowed to answer student questions. At least one practice station is maintained and staffed during the testing period. Time is structured so that students always have an assigned activity. King County classes have varied in size from 3 students and 1 instructor to 50 students and 7 instructors. It is imperative that sufficient equipment be available to allow students plenty of practice and review time with the device.

Instructor Qualifications and Precourse Meeting Agenda

Physician program medical director. The medical director should present some portion of the didactic lecture of the class and has final say on the student's final testing skills.

Program coordinator. This person delivers the didactic sections not covered by the medical director, coordinates instructors, and assigns tasks for class demonstrations and small-group teaching. The coordinator assembles all equipment and checks to be sure that all instructors are trained in the skills and are aware of class objectives. They also remain available as much as possible to answer student questions concerning the program and/or skills.

Practical instructors. In King County these instructors have been experienced EMT-D personnel who were also CPR instructors. They have helped develop the practical portions of the class and know the devices and the program well enough to answer most questions that arise. Prior to each class they review and perform the standing orders for program coordinator to assure uniform teaching in the class:

Introduction and paperwork
Introductory lecture by physician medical director
Demonstration of the AED/SAED in action
Introduction to the components of the defibrillator
Standing orders introduction and practical group session
Questions and answers

Class 1: Introduction to Automatic Defibrillation—Back from the Jaws of Death

Time	Elapsed	
:15		Introduction and paperwork
:15	:30	Introductory comments from medical director
:15	:45	Demonstration 1: the standing orders
:15	1:00	Demonstration 2: the defibrillator
:15	1:15	Demonstration 3: cardiac arrest!
:45	2:00	Small-group practice: using a defibrillator
:15	2:15	Whole-class question-and-answer session

Class 1: Introduction to Automatic Defibrillation

Time Required	Contents	Instructor Notes
:15 (:15)	1. *Introduction and paperwork* a. Attendance roll, instructors introduced b. Program prerequisites c. Student information package distributed d. Orientation to information packages: (1) Description of contents (2) Requirements for EMT-D authorization (3) Course objectives	Program coordinator should introduce self and instructors. An attendance roll should be circulated while the program prerequisites are reviewed. The student package should be handed out and the contents described. Emphasize the packet as the source of answers to many questions. Request that the students save their questions until the time allotted for questions, and that many questions will be answered during the course of the program. The sheet in the student package that describes the course objectives should be reviewed.
:15 (:30)	2. *Introductory lecture: sudden cardiac death and the new breed of rescuers* a. Brief review of relevant cardiac anatomy and electrophysiology b. Importance of early defibrillation c. Limitations of CPR d. Brief history of sudden cardiac death e. The dying heart f. What defibrillation and a defibrillator are g. What an automatic defibrillator is h. Signs of an impending heart attack i. The cure for sudden death: back to the basics plus defibrillation (1) Careful assessment	The program *medical director* is encouraged to deliver this brief talk if possible. A possible outline for the first is suggested above. It is extremely helpful for the rescuers to observe the interest and support of the medical director, and to hear the medical director emphasize the value of the skill of defibrillation.

Class 1: Introduction to Automatic Defibrillation (*cont.*)

Time Required	Contents	Instructor Notes
	(2) Speedy treatment (3) Controlled scene (4) Good CPR (5) Rapid defibrillation (6) Early advanced life support	
Optional/Required (May take up to 1:00)	3. *CPR and ventilation skill practical review* a. One-person CPR b. Two-person CPR c. Ventilation adjuncts	EMT-Ds and first responders must be able to perform competent one- and two-person CPR and be proficient in the recommended ventilation adjuncts. Programs can either assume competency in these areas as a prerequisite to the class, or test these skills prior to or as part of the initial EMT-D class. Emphasize one-person CPR if most units respond with only two-person teams.
:15 (:45)	4. *Demonstration 1: standing orders* *DON'T BE LATE–DEFIBRILLATE!* a. *Define:* (1) Standing orders (2) Medical control b. Demonstration of actual defibrillation and standing orders. Rhythm is ventricular fibrillation: (1) Three shocks to ventricular fibrillation. (2) Converts to normal sinus rhythm with a pulse (a perfusing rhythm). (3) Blood pressure is 60 mmHg (CPR stops). (4) Patient does not resume respirations. (5) Ventilation support provided.	Two instructors demonstrate the standing orders in front of the class. Another instructor narrate their activities. They use a defibrillator, a simulator, and a resuscitation manikin. One instructor is the defibrillation technician and the other performs CPR. The simulator produces a ventricular fibrillation tracing for the defibrillator. One instructor provides commentary on the demonstration.

Time	Content	Notes
:15 (1:00)	5. *Demonstration 2: orientation to the defibrillator.* All parts of the defibrillator and its supportive equipment are described. The instructor displays an AED or SAS in front of the class. Controls should be described in the sequence in which they will be used in a cardiac arrest.	Encourage students to move so that they can see the demonstration clearly. The defibrillator is placed on a table for easy viewing. The charging unit and simulator are also displayed. All parts of the device are displayed and their use defined. The defibrillator's disposable items are described. The defibrillator pads are placed on a student volunteer or a manikin that has been prepared with Armoral. This is the time to discuss machine maintenance and safety issues.
:15 (1:15)	6. *Demonstration 3: cardiac arrest!* Demonstration of these cardiac arrest scenarios: a. The rhythm is ventricular fibrillation; the patient gets one shock and regains a pulse. b. The rhythm is ventricular fibrillation; the patient gets two shocks and does not regain a pulse. c. The rhythm is asystole; the patient gets no shocks. d. The patient is a conscious patient who arrests during transport to the hospital. The patient gets four shocks and regains a rhythm.	
	Break into small groups.	
:45 (2:00)	7. *Small-group practical:* Presentation of a step-by-step description of how to use an AED in a cardiac arrest. During this time the students practice the various scenarios and evaluate each others' performance.	Class breaks into small groups with no more than six students per instructor. See the equipment list for items needed in each teaching station. During this hour each student should have the opportunity to practice with the defibrillator at least four times. Talk the students through each step. Encourage questions from the students at all times. The instructor comments on each of the topics to the left during this session.

Class 1: Introduction to Automatic Defibrillation (*cont.*)

Time Required	Contents	Instructor Notes
	a. *The EMT roles at the scene.* Upon arrival at the scene, one EMT is the defibrillation technician, who operates the AED and assumes control of the scene. The other EMT begins basic life support. The instructors will stress the importance of defining these roles before arrival at the scene. b. *Scene control.* Responsibility for directing the medical treatment of the patient rests with the defibrillation technician. This is especially true when the patient must be clear of all contact with people. c. *Rapid defibrillation.* Rapid defibrillation should be performed within 90 seconds of the defibrillator touching the floor next to the patient. d. *The high priority of defibrillation.* No other activities, including setting up oxygen delivery systems, suction equipment, advanced airway procedures, IVs, or mechanical CPR devices should take precedence over defibrillation.	
	Next in the small-group practical the instructors present all details necessary for successful operation of the AED/SAED in a cardiac arrest. These steps and details are supplied below. This material will also be reviewed during the small-group practical in class 2.	
	(1) *Defibrillator placement.* Place the AED device close to the patient's left ear and perform the defibrillation protocols from the left side of the patient.	Better access to the defibrillator controls and placement of the defibrillatory pads on the chest is achieved with the AED and the defibrillator

Timing for performance testing begins when the defibrillator is set down.	technician in these positions. This may not, however, be possible in all clinical situations. Discuss alternatives.
(2) *Power control.* Turn the power ON and make sure that the tape recorder is running.	Remind the students that one EMT is starting CPR while the defibrillation technician is preparing the AED to assess the rhythm and defibrillate if ventricular fibrillation is present. It is the defibrillation technician's responsibility to assure that adequate CPR is performed.
(3) *Narration begins.* The EMT/first responder should: • Identify herself or himself and the responding EMS unit. • Briefly describe the clinical situation. • Report each step while proceeding through the standing orders. • State whether shocks are delivered. • Continue to provide explanatory comments on actions, decisions to transport, problems, and so on.	Be prepared to provide several example narrations during this demonstration of the equipment. Verbal reports can be too short, with insufficient information provided, or too long, with distraction from the performance of the defibrillation protocols.
(4) *Defibrillatory chest pad placement.* The adhesive defibrillatory chest pads are opened and attached to a manikin in the proper locations: • *White or sternum pad* to the right border of the sternum, with the top edge just touching the bottom of the clavicle • *Red or apex pad* to the left lower ribs, at the anterior axillary line	Demonstrate a NO CONTACT signal caused by improper placement of the pads. Demonstrate how the person doing CPR must briefly move their hands to achieve proper pad placement. Review how to open the packaging for the adhesive pads. Discuss some problems that might occur with defibrillatory pad placement.
(5) *Attach defibrillator cables to the adhesive pads.* Manufacturer instructions may vary on this point. Some recommend attachment of the defibrillator cables to the adhesive pads prior to placement on the patient's chest.	Spend some time to make sure that each student knows exactly how to open the adhesive pad package, properly attach the pads to the correct locations on the patient, and correctly attach the defibrillator cables to the adhesive pads.

Class 1: Introduction to Automatic Defibrillation (*cont.*)

Time Required	Contents	Instructor Notes
	Note: The exact details of rhythm analysis and shock delivery will vary with the brand of AED/SAED.	
	(6) *Begin rhythm analysis.* Press the analysis control switch on the AED/SAED. The switch may be labeled AUTOMATIC/MANUAL or ANALYZE, depending on the brand of AED/SAED. Verify that everyone is clear of the patient. If a chart recorder is available, or if there is a separate control for the tape recorder, make sure that they are running.	Several brands of AED/SAEDs require that several questions be answered by the operator by pushing YES or NO switches on a liquid-crystal display screen. These questions must be answered before the device will continue with assessment.
	(7) *Assessment.* Everyone must remain clear of the patient while assessment is in progress. Assessment take no more than 15 to 20 seconds, depending on the brand of AED/SAED. Operators should count to 15 slowly and out loud during the assessment periods. If by the count of 15 the device has not delivered a shock or has indicated that a shock was not advised, resume CPR. The devices will indicate that charging is underway with a tone, voice-synthesized message, or light indicators. Physical motion will cause false interpretation.	

	(8) *Deliver countershocks.* Fully automatic AEDs will deliver countershocks without additional actions from the operator. For shock advisory devices, a message such as "shock advised" or "shock now" will be presented to the operator from either a liquid-crystal display or a voice synthesizer. (9) *Resume CPR.* Perform one to four cycles of compressions and ventilations, depending on the local standing orders. This may require removing the device from the automatic or analysis mode. (10) *Repeat rhythm assessment and shock delivery.* Standing orders will vary on the number of repeat countershocks and rhythm assessment periods. The NASEMSTC National Standards recommends: three consecutive shocks 15 seconds of CPR three consecutive shocks	Standing orders will vary among emergency systems. In general, three consecutive shocks will be delivered without interruption if the rhythm is persistent ventricular fibrillation.
10 minutes	8. *Class summary.* Entire class regroups for a summary and a time for questions and answers.	The medical director or program coordinator is in charge of this session. If possible, equipment should be made available for students who wish to practice between the classes.

Class 2: Putting It All Together

Time required	Total elapsed	
:30		Medical control and the EMT/first responder
:15	:45	Troubleshooting the device
1:00	1:45	Small-group practice
:30–?	2:15–?	Written and practical testing

Class 2: Putting It All Together

Time Required	Contents

:30 (:30)

1. *Medical control and the EMT/first responder.* This lecture is preferably given by the program medical director. These areas should be reviewed:
   - a. Review the standing orders and field protocols.
   - b. Define event documentation. The medical director defines his or her expectations about:
     - (1) The voice narration.
     - (2) The written run report.
     - (3) The paper ECG strip if the particular device provides one.
     - (4) How to contact the program medical director and program coordinator about a specific case.
   - c. Define the program requirement for skill maintenance.
   - d. Review postshock care of the cardiac arrest patient:
     - (1) When to stop CPR (for a blood pressure with a diastolic blood pressure 60 mmHg).
     - (2) Airway maintenance adjuncts and when to use each one in the protocols.
     - (3) Getting the patient ready for transport. Never allow the AED/SAED to assess the patient's rhythm while the vehicle is moving.

:15 (:45)

2. *Troubleshooting the device, and covering special circumstances.* Describe the proper procedure for these possibilities:
   - a. Patient electrode contact problems. Diaphoretic patients need to be dried with whatever is available. The rescuers must be prepared with extra adhesive pads.
   - b. Nitro paste patches on the patient. Place the pads away from these patches, and remove the paste with a 4 × 4 gauze pad or whatever is available.
   - c. Pacemaker implanted in the patient's skin. Place the pad approximately 5 inches from this site.
   - d. Scene control.
   - e. Hazards: water, swimming pools, bath tubs, and so on.

Class 2: Putting It All Together ***(cont.)***

Time Required	Contents
	f. Clearing the patient from all human contact during the AED/SAED assessment period. Be especially careful with bystanders who have been helping with CPR, since they may not be familiar with your procedures.
1:00 (1:45)	3. *Small-group practice time.* This time is reserved for students to practice various events that may occur in the field. The instructors give the two-person EMT/first responder teams several scenarios during which they perform the protocols. The instructors should vary the clinical situations, the rhythms, and the patient responses. During this session the instructors should have a perception of which students are proficient with the skills and which students will need more practice prior to testing.
	Some scenarios are presented: ventricular fibrillation that requires six shocks, that converts to asystole after shock, and that converts to a perfusing rhythm after shock; one example of artifact troubleshooting; asystole as the initial rhythm; refibrillation after a perfusing rhythm; patients that have to be moved from one location to another; and cardiac arrest both during transport and in a doctor's office.
	4. *Testing.* The entire class reconvenes to take the written test. One instructor is available for questions about the test. The criterion for successful passage of the practical testing is whether or not defibrillatory shocks would be delivered to patients in ventricular fibrillation safely, rapidly, and competently. Both the practical testing stations *and* the skill practice station should remain available (maximum of three tries at the practical examination) until everyone has passed.